UNITARY
Caring Science

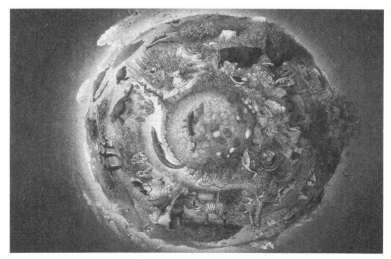

Frontispiece: Unitary Caring Science: Philosophy and Praxis

Please visit https://www.watsoncaringscience.org/freegift to receive four free videos. Each one is selected specifically for additional understandings of Unitary Caring Science: education, teaching, and personal-inspirational meditation.

The following videos are accessed through private links to Jean's Vimeo account.

Education/Teachings

1) **Jean "End Notes" closing keynote video**: Unitary Caring Science–2016 Boston Conference; the first joint conference of the IAHC-SRS (International Association of Human Caring and the Society of Rogerian Scholars).

2) **Overview of Human Caring**: a teaching summary of caring science theory as a guide to practice.

Meditation/Blessings

1) Blessing meditation for nurses
2) Personal meditation

The classic *Caring Moment* audio will continue to be available for free. Please complete the online form to receive a confirmation email to access the videos.

UNITARY
Caring Science
The Philosophy and
Praxis of Nursing

Jean Watson
PhD, RN, AHN-BC, FAAN

Living Legend AAN
WWW.WATSONCARINGSCIENCE.ORG
JEAN@WATSONCARINGSCIENCE.ORG

Founder-Director Watson Caring Science Institute

Distinguished Professor/Dean Emerita
UNIVERSITY OF COLORADO DENVER,
COLLEGE OF NURSING

UNIVERSITY PRESS OF COLORADO
Louisville

Published by the University Press of Colorado
245 Century Circle, Suite 202
Louisville, Colorado 80027

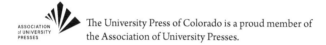 The University Press of Colorado is a proud member of
the Association of University Presses.

The University Press of Colorado is a cooperative publishing enterprise supported, in part, by Adams State College, Colorado State University, Fort Lewis College, Mesa State College, Metropolitan State College of Denver, University of Colorado, University of Northern Colorado, and Western State College of Colorado.

∞ The paper used in this publication meets the minimum requirements of the American National Standard for Information Sciences—Permanence of Paper for Printed Library Materials. ANSI Z39.48-1992

ISBN: 978-1-60732-755-4 (paperback)
ISBN: 978-1-60732-756-1 (ebook)
DOI: https://doi.org/10.5876/9781607327561

Library of Congress Cataloging-in-Publication Data

Names: Watson, Jean, 1940– author.
Title: Unitary caring science : philosophy and praxis of nursing / Jean Watson.
Description: Boulder : University Press of Colorado, [2018]
Identifiers: LCCN 2018017431| ISBN 9781607327554 (pbk.) | ISBN 9781607327561 (ebook)
Subjects: LCSH: Nursing—Philosophy. | Holistic nursing. | Nursing models. | Nursing ethics. | Nursing—Practice. | Caring—Philosophy.
Classification: LCC RT84.5 .W38 2018 | DDC 610.7301—dc23
LC record available at https://lccn.loc.gov/2018017431

Dedication

This book is dedicated, as always, to my precious family—daughters Jennifer and Julie and grandchildren Demitri, Alma, and Theo Ervedosa and Gabriel and Joseph Willis.

This book represents an evolution of caring science theory and contributes to an archive of scholarly work that has evolved over the past forty years. It is hoped that the work has had an impact on and maybe even become imprinted in and inspired others with heart-to-heart connections, based on my career experiences, publications, worldwide speaking, consulting, teaching, researching, and administrating with others. This continuing work is motivated by a commitment to develop a distinct specific caring philosophy (and theory of transpersonal caring) for unitary science and praxis as moral practice, informed by the discipline and framed as Unitary Caring Science. It is therefore a living process of evolving Caritas toward more complexity, more enlightenment for sustaining and moving human consciousness toward Infinite Divine Love as the basis for all healing.

This book is further dedicated to the thousands, if not millions, of nurses touched by the writings, teachings, and seminars, as well as workshops in human caring theory and caring science, I have offered around the world. It honors those many others who have inspired, inspirited, informed, and expanded my ongoing evolution in my personal and professional growth. Every travel encounter around the world has given me more courage, affirmation, and confidence to continue to advance caring science in the unitary field for our work and our world. Each encounter reminds us—society and the public—of nursing's global, universal, timeless, and enduring moral covenant with humanity: to sustain and preserve human caring, healing, and health for all.

Students and colleagues around the world continue to inspire and inform me about the deeper nature of this work and its potential for generating love and caring globally, opening new horizons for caring, healing, and peace in the world.

I always am learning from inspirited others who explore nursing theory as a living presence in transforming their personal and professional lives and likewise mine.

I also remind everyone: I write and teach what I am learning, needing continually to learn. Through my ongoing questioning, inner quests, and intellectual-spiritual pursuits, perhaps I am finding the answers to my own rhetorical questions. However, you, the reader, will know what you need to learn only if you pursue your personal enduring questions. I trust that this work, in some small way, helps you to know and follow your own way, through your own pursuits, in this magnificent, ancient, noble, and evolving field of nursing.

Side Note

The focus of this work is not for every nurse but for the students, faculty, scholars, and researchers who are dedicated to furthering the development of nursing as a distinct discipline and profession of Unitary Caring Science, integrating caring-healing practices into education, practice, research, and administrative leadership policies, principles, and practices and into their daily lives. This book is for the Caritas Nurse®, or those Caritas Practitioners, nursing scholars, educators, faculty, and students who are on the journey toward the deeper caring-healing dimensions of life and are on a personal-professional path of authenticity and evolution of consciousness, bringing universals of Love, Energy, Spirit, Infinity of Purpose, and Meaning back into their lives and their life's work in the world. This work also serves as a disciplinary foundation for nursing to mature at a higher level of evolution so it can fulfill its mission to humanity. For scholars and educators, this work serves as a guide to new theories and emerging research traditions for new forms of Unitary Caring Science inquiry, and it serves as a philosophical guide to knowledge development and advanced praxis.

This work serves as a continuing, evolving message to the next generation of nurses and health scholars, clinicians, and practitioners engaged in and committed to a unitary worldview of Caritas knowledge, allowing the discipline of nursing to inform education, practice, and inquiry within an evolved, ethical cosmology of oneness of all.

Contents

CONTENTS

Acknowledgments

I thank Watson Caring Science Institute (WCSI), the remarkable WCSI faculty associates who have partnered with me on this journey into caring science/unitary caring science. I am touched by WCSI board members, past and current, and devoted colleagues who continue to live and embrace this work in their lifework. I offer special gratitude to Ronald Lesinski, founding president of WCSI, who for the past ten years has sustained his belief in and support of this work and me—traveling, consulting, videotaping me, and facilitating my presentations and presence through almost monthly global presentations on different continents and in countries with diverse cultures. I also continue to be grateful for Barbara Hope and Don Gaiti and the late Jeremy Geffen, MD, for their early sustained support for WCSI and for me personally.

My appreciation is extended to Darrin Pratt and the University Press of Colorado for their continuing interest and support in keeping this original work alive and moving forward, evolving into the future for a new generation of faculty, students, and practitioners. This book advances, expands, and supplements the original publications on caring science, helping to sustain caring-healing philosophical values, moral ideals, passion, intellectual, experiential growth, and consciousness evolution. It is through evolutionary turns that we bring more clarity to the discipline of nursing, helping to sustain humanity and universals of human caring, healing, and peace in our work and our world. All of this unfolding results in an expanded unitary worldview, grounded in the Ethic of Belonging explicated through a unitary caring science disciplinary lens, underpinned by the philosophy and ontology of cosmic love. This convergence of caring science and cosmic universal energy of love serves as the disciplinary lens for unitary caring praxis—practice that is morally guided by a unitary, even quantum worldview of oneness, of connectedness of practice, with congruence between and among core philosophy, values, ethics, ontology, theory, knowledge, and approaches to knowledge development for human caring-healing professional practices. These practices within the disciplinary structure are manifest through ten Caritas-(Veritas) processes; these core processes provide a moral as well as a theoretical language for the sacred living universals of human caring, contributing to healing and even peace in our world.

Historical Backdrop: Other Books

Here I review my other books on transpersonal caring theory and caring science that have influenced the field. Some of them have been translated into at least nine languages. The other major theory-based books on caring that followed the original 1979 book include:

- *Nursing: Human Science and Human Care: A Theory of Nursing* (1985). East Norwich, CT: Appleton-Century-Crofts. Reprinted/republished (1988). New York: National League for Nursing. Reprinted/republished (1999). Sudbury, MA: Jones and Bartlett.

- *Postmodern Nursing and Beyond* (1999). Edinburgh, Scotland: Churchill-Livingstone. Reprinted/republished New York: Elsevier. Reprinted (2011). Boulder, CO: Watson Caring Science Institute. www.watsoncaringscience.org.
- *Assessing and Measuring Caring in Nursing and Health Science* (ed.) (2002) (revised 2008). New York: Springer (AJN Book of the Year award).
- *Caring Science as Sacred Science* (2005). Philadelphia: F. A. Davis (AJN Book of the Year award).
- *Caring Science: Mindful Practice* (2012). New York: Springer. (K. Sitzman and J. Watson).
- *Global Caring Literacy* (2016). New York: Springer. (S. Lee, P. Palmieri, and J. Watson).
- Rosa, W., S. Horton-Deutsch, and J. Watson (eds.) (2018, in process). *Handbook of Caring Science*. New York: Springer.

Please see the Watson Caring Science Institute website: www.watsoncaringscience.org, https://www.watsoncaringscience.org/jean-bio/publications/ for complete citations of all books, publications, videos, meditations, presentations, and teachings.

Preface

Opening

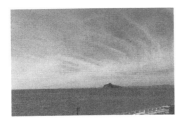
Bahia, Mexico

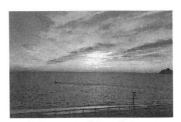
Bahia sunset—inspiring writing

I return to the quiet of Bahia, Mexico, my sanctuary space, where I can be still and quiet the busy mind and the busyness of the outer world. The moon is half full, leaving space for filling up and running over, creating lunar openness for heartfelt reflections of gratitude as I take an evening walk on this Friday, January 6, 2017.

The original work (1979) presented a human caring framework as the foundation, the soul, the core and essence of nursing as a discipline and a profession. The 2008 2nd revised edition both summarized and expanded the entire original work: *Nursing: The Philosophy and Science of Caring.*

I now offer a new book, building upon earlier work but bringing another revolution/evolution in my personal/professional queries and quests as well as in advancing a better understanding of human caring-healing and health for our world. Also, the present work helps anchor caring science and, in turn, unitary caring science as a unitary transformative worldview. This, in turn, contributes to a maturing of the discipline of nursing. This maturing invites a converging unitary disciplinary worldview that underpins nursing theories, ethics, ontology, and epistemologies—critiquing what counts as knowledge. Thus the unitary discipline worldview of nursing and unitary caring serves as a guide to inform education, practice, research, forms of inquiry, administration, and policy directions for healthcare. The result is a unitary caring science philosophy and praxis.

Being here, in the quiet of Mexico, is like a new wave upon the shore, revealing the oceanic sea-of-thinking that still runs through my life career and my collected works on caring. I am continually writing, teaching, traveling, experiencing, learning, and pondering ideas from nurses around the globe. I seek what I need to learn.

Here in Mexico, I love placing myself near the magnetic rhythm, the pull of the sea. I lose myself. My mood gets silent, quiet, and in harmony with the tide and waves as I watch them rising up and crashing/spilling on to the shoreline. Some are soft and gentle, others are deep whitecaps that come from far out in the depths of Mar de Cortez. So, nature washes over me, cleansing out the busy schedule prior to being here.

Here I create open space between the waves, like the pause between drumbeats, opening and receptive to what is emerging. Or, open to what wants to emerge, from the deep inner sea of my experiences around the globe over the past decade, since my last book.

Not knowing how this book will unfold but open to its emergence, I invite others to enter and follow my path into the future. At this moment I am openly anticipatory as this journey takes me forward. What has already emerged is a new title: *Unitary Caring Science: Philosophy and Praxis of Nursing.*

Unitary caring science as both philosophy and praxis begins with an evolved worldview of oneness and connections of all; it involves being conscious, intentional, and authentically present; open to compassion, mercy, gentleness, loving-kindness, and equanimity toward and with self before any of us can offer compassionate caring to others. It requires an understanding that how one is with oneself affects how one is with others and, in turn, affects the whole; also, how one is with others affects how one is with oneself and affects the whole. This is a lifetime journey.

As Rumi reminded us:

It doesn't matter that you've broken
Your vow a thousand times, still
Come, and yet again, come.
Don't pretend to know
Something you haven't experienced.

We cannot know caring unless we have learned it from within, for our self, with our self, and with others—within a relational worldview. Human caring begins with a love of self and other, of humanity and all living things—opening and welcoming the immanent and transcendent, the subtle, radiant, shadow-and-light vicissitudes of experiences of embodied living, dying, growing, changing, evolving; honoring with reverence the mystery, miracles, paradoxes, unknowns, the impermanence of changes while still actively, joyfully participating in all of it: the pain, the joy, and everything, believing in and allowing for miracles.

Thus, to open and enter this living process of unitary caring science philosophy and praxis, I invite you again to engage in a centering mindful process, a reflective pause, and a contemplative meditation:

First, Just Pause—Empty Out

- Take a deep renewing breath. Fall into your heart; open your heart to this now, this breath of life. Listen quietly to your silent inner voice; why are you here? Why are you in nursing?
- In this quiet inner space, bow with simple gratitude and humility for your life and all your blessings, even if you feel dispirited. In this silence conjure an awakening feeling, sensing and knowing

that your life is sacred and full of awe and mystery. Let yourself feel that wherever you are, you are on holy ground.

• Breathe in this holy connection, which is closer than breath itself.

• From this quiet inner sacred place, release it all to the universe; embrace the wonder of life's gifts and open to your own awakening to Universal Love, knowing you are loved and are Love.

This work gathers up an expanded awareness and understanding of unitary caring science, gleaned from nurses all over the world. Their call is my call: to return to one's inner sacred heart-core; to reconnect with the timeless collective foundation and the very soul of this ancient, pioneering, and noble profession of human caring–healing–health for all. This call is also a call for nursing to mature as a distinct caring-healing discipline, grounded in a unitary worldview that is worthy of its phenomena of wholeness, evolving consciousness, oneness, and caring. This call acknowledges human caring as a serious moral, ethical, ontological, epistemological, practical praxis endeavor, not to be taken for granted. Thus, if caring science is not pursued within a distinct disciplinary unitary worldview, the discipline may not survive; the profession may be reduced to being subsumed under other disciplines and nurses to practice as very good technicians within a totally transformed unitary worldview of science and medicine. We are entering a quantum universe that we cannot ignore, inviting an awakening for all of humanity if we are to survive.

Translating Our Call to Caring Service to Unitary Caring Science

To return to our united global call for human caring–healing–health—we cannot take it for granted. It requires serious attention to and focused intention on global sacred activism for humanity and planet earth. As noted, this call is a serious moral, ethical, epistemological, ontological, philosophical endeavor, a serious concrete practical endeavor. It is incumbent upon the discipline of nursing to give credible voice to another view of science, another view of human caring, healing, health as part of the sacred circle of life, connecting with the universal cosmic source of Love that unites rather than separates. This shift is beyond Western medical science and beyond nursing as we have known it. This work offers an evolved, intellectual, ethical, and experiential foundation and orientation toward Unitary Caring Science as the foundation for unitary caring praxis, to honor the true nature of what nursing has to offer to humanity. It also reflects the changing, evolving, expanding unitary view of our humanity, our world, our planet, our reality.

Unitary caring science awakens humans and science to an evolved worldview, a cosmology of one Humanity, one Heart, one World, one Planet Earth on which we all reside. There is no separate world; there are no humans separate from us, from each other; there are no humans living separately from Planet Earth, from each other. We are all one within the cosmic universal field of life energy. While this book builds upon caring science, it evolves toward unitary caring science. Once one places the phenomena of wholeness, energy, and caring-healing and evolving consciousness within a unitary worldview, it has to end up as unitary caring science.

This work provides a distinct focus for the discipline of nursing for caring and healing; it provides a moral, ethical, philosophical, ontological, and knowledge foundation, guiding nursing practice, moving from practice-for-institutional-practice's sake to praxis—that is, informed moral practice guided by our core timeless values, knowledge, unitary worldview, consciousness, unitary connections, thus, our discipline's worldview, a love of humanity and human existence in all its complexities and unknowns. Caring science and unitary caring science invite concepts and phenomena that dwell and believe in Ambiguity, Angels, Appreciation, Ancestors, Artistry, and Activism—Sacred Activism. Unitary caring science incorporates metaphysical, non-physical/physical as one and the same. The ten Caritas Processes of the Transpersonal Theory of Human Caring continue to offer a universal language so that nurses can name, "see,"

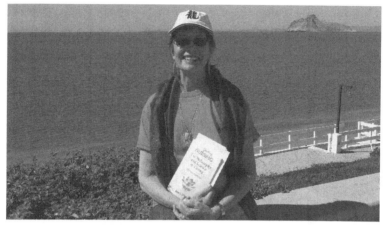

Jean Watson in Bahia, Mar de Cortez, Mexico. Photo by Ronald Lesinski.

and live Caritas in our world. Caritas-Veritas brings a new dimension to moral literacy as a guide to affirming and sustaining the timeless gift nursing praxis offers to our world.

This book can be read straightforwardly or wherever within it you happen to turn. It is at once linear, sequential, and non-linear—so let it take you where you are drawn, to enter and follow the evolution and emergent quality of this work. Let yourself experience a transpersonal moment as you enter.

Transpersonal caring moments capture the "eternal now" of the moment—transcending time, space, and physicality; they endure throughout our lives. Sometimes I tell myself (as my poet friend Marilyn Krysl says), "I am standing still and moving at the speed of light." As we reenter nursing and its evolving maturity, we are uniting with over 20 million nurses and midwives on the planet and more than 7 billion people—all crying out for healing in some way, to be embraced with love and knowledgeable human caring connections. In small and grand ways, transpersonal caring is one with the unitary field, touching all of humanity. Therefore, I hope these ideas touch you and your heart with inner knowing.

My hope is that this evolving work will contribute to the discipline of nursing, to y/our awakening to wisdom and compassion.

Love and caring-healing, moral-ethical, committed values are world-view practices that are essential to sustain the enduring and timeless gift of self to others. I thank you for being Y O U; we are co-creating a new world, even if we are not aware of it.

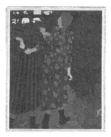

Young Girls Walking
by Edouard Vuillard, ca. 1891

Interlude Continuing (*revised from Watson 2008, xxi*)

You/We who do not know the future of nursing and healthcare
We/You who know too much of the past
Now step into new space
You/We create new options
Envision new hopes
And possibilities not yet dreamt of—
Vibrating possibilities
Waiting to unfold for humanity, for health, for healing, for peace,
For Being-Doing-Becoming Caritas in a new tune.
Learning a new song—
A new sound, a new rhythm, a new Voice
Opening to that which might be, not conforming to what already is
And which no longer serves
Self, System, Society.
You/We the old and new
As you encounter anyone who tells you
Nursing is less than what you know and believe,
Bless them and turn away.
If what anyone tells you is fear-based, limited, or limiting,
Also bless them and turn away.
Turn toward Love and Caritas from your own deep self.
You, aligned with your higher Source, are the source of your own
    power and possibilities.

Background

Personal Pause

> We, as nursing and health professionals, know that when we step
> into the theories and philosophies of human caring, we step into a
> deep ethic and life practice that connects us with the heart of our
> humanity, of healing the whole; it is here in this connection that we
> touch the mystery of inner and outer peace that unites humanity
> across time and space around the world.
>
> JEAN WATSON

I enter/reenter this work from here in Mexico, where I take time
out/time in to go inward to write from the inner space inspired by
nature and the sea. I am a Cancer astrological water sign, so it nour-
ishes me to be here in this quiet, peaceful space. If you look at the
photo you can see the sea in the background, which is my view from
my writing place. There in the foreground is a copy of the 2008 revised edition of the "lotus" book.

Also, if you had more personal information about me and looked
more closely, you would recognize the two beautiful healing stones

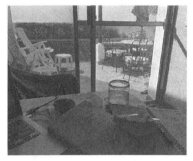 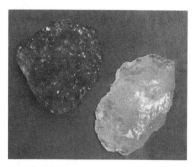

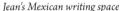

Jean's Mexican writing space   *Brazilian healing stones*

on my little desk. One is citrine, referred to as a joyful stone, combating negative energy and manifesting a positive field. The other is rose quartz, the love, heart energy stone that generates mental harmony and love for self/others.

The stones depicted here are from the famous, more than twenty-year-old village, Abadiania, Casa de Dom Inacio, outside Brasilia, Brazil; this is the World Spiritual Healing Center site of St. John of God, where millions of miraculous healings have occurred. I was privileged to experience this center through one of my graduate students in Brazil, Amarry Morbeck. Both stones carry the vibrational healing energy from that site, which I carried back from my visit there in November 2016.

In the photo the reader has a glimpse of my personal workspace, simple and sparse. It is being in such an isolated, simple space with nature and sea that I am nourished and freed. Also, it is a full moon, January 11, 2017, so the atmosphere is alive with the vibrancy of high energy. The tide is much farther out than I have ever seen in more than thirty years of coming to this little sanctuary, first with family, then with grandchildren, and now for myself.

I connect with Anne Morrow Lindbergh and her sea, sand, and seashells as *gifts from the sea*. Over the years I have changed the way I receive "gifts from the sea"; rather than collect shells, as before, I now just appreciate them and try to recognize the angel wings, chamber nautilus, turkey feet, cowrie, whelks, Scotch Bonnet, calico scallop,

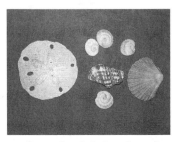

Small view of my "gifts from the sea."

the occasional treasure of a sand dollar, and others, including little button swirls.

(I confess that I still pick up the little pearl button shells. I have them in all my pockets and purses. I keep them as little touchstones, as reminders of the sea and also as a reminder of the great circle of life. Everything is a circle—even in nature).

Now, I come to the sea for walking and writing but also for simple time out/time in. A place and a time to empty out, to pause, to learn, to bow to mystery, to live my own writing.

UNITARY
Caring Science

Part One

CHAPTER ONE

The Philosophy of Science

*Starting Point/Inverting the Paradigm**

STARTING POINT: *the starting point will dictate where you end up.*

INVERTING THE PARADIGM

Behind everything physical in the world lies the unseen substance of Spirit . . . God is the unseen source and substance of everything that exists.

DAILY WORD, JANUARY 8, 2017, 21

A more complete study of the movements of the world will oblige us, little by little, to turn it upside down.

PIERRE TEILHARD DE CHARDIN 1955, 43

INVERTING THE PARADIGM

- From physical to non-physical—metaphysical; to spiritual— open to infinity

---

* This chapter is heavily adapted from J. Watson, M. Smith, and R. Cowling, "Unitary Caring Science: Disciplinary Evolution of Nursing," in W. Rosa, S. Horton-Deutsch, and J. Watson, eds., *Handbook of Caring Science* (New York: Springer, 2018 [in press]).

- From treatment and curing to caring-healing
- From caring as a means to an end to an end in and of itself—a highest ethical ideal for society, for a moral community
- From dense, medicalized language to evocative Caritas-Veritas language
- From separatist ontology to unitary-relational ontology
- From particulate to interactive to unitary transformative paradigm thinking
- From 'consciousness'—'residing-in-the-body physical'—to 'non-local consciousness' to body residing in infinite field of universal consciousness—Cosmic Love
- From 'Epistemology as Ethic' to 'Ethic of Belonging'
- From low-vibration human consciousness actions to higher vibration of an evolved global human heart/consciousness connection
- From fear-based Ego living to Trust—Truth-Love—Beauty living Caritas-Veritas
- From medical-clinicalized views of humanity to reverential respect for one humanity—one world, one heart, one planet earth
- From institutional technical medical cure practices to Unitary Caring Science Praxis.

Science is all a tall story we tell ourselves.

W. H. AUDEN

Thomas Berry (1988) wrote about how we are searching for a New Story within which we find a sense of life purpose, a guide to education, an understanding of our suffering, and impetus for energized action—what Andrew Harvey (2009) refers to as "sacred activism." It is becoming increasingly obvious that the Old Story of science and medical science, as our starting point for society and life, has become fragmented and nonfunctional. Unitary caring science offers a New Story for science and our existence, if not our survival.

In a conventional medical science mind-set, caring has been seen as a means to an end, a curing end—an end, often at all costs, emotionally, psychologically, medically, spiritually. When we invert the paradigm and reexamine human caring as a serious endeavor, we can acknowledge that, yes, caring contributes to curing. However, by turning the paradigm upside down, we position human caring as an end in and of itself, not just a means to a medical-cure end. Indeed, by inverting the paradigm, we place human caring as the highest ethical ideal we can offer society and humanity.*

In the world of science, Willis Harman (1999) proposed another way for us to turn the scientific paradigm upside down. For example, he noted that in the conventional world of Western science we have what he called "the downward causation" model of science, whereby if we invert it we can consider an upward causation model of science. That is, rather than focus on smaller and smaller separate parts, we can consider moving upward to more complex explanatory models that accommodate more information and higher-level abstraction, including spirit and spiritual science, the science of consciousness.

Praxis of unitary caring science makes explicit the underlying values, ethics, as part of the entire single unitary field of human-earth-universe. It moves the Caritas Processes of Praxis to embrace Veritas, the Latin word for truth, beauty, love, goodness, restoring the moral component within the full meaning of Praxis. Caritas and Veritas combine in unitary caring science, returning nursing to its underlying purity and purpose of basic goodness. These underlying values are needed today to offer a New Story of science and actions that can help sustain our humanity and planet earth.

As part of the New Story of unity and human-universe caring, Thomas Berry's (1988) "New Story" is a call to honor and embrace the universe itself as the basic value, the most profound primary sacred community on the planet. Indeed, he proclaimed that "all human activities, all professions, all programs and institutions must henceforth be judged primarily by the extent [to which] they

---

* This ethical ideal was influenced by philosopher Sally Gadow.

inhabit, ignore or foster a mutually enhancing human-earth relation as one" (Melange 2009).

> If we encourage [them] to enter the profession without making any conditions as to the way in which the professions are to be practiced ... shall we be encouraging the very qualities we wish to prevent? War, non-caring, violence ...
>
> Shall we swear that the professions in the future shall be practiced so that they lead to a different song and a different conclusion?
>
> VIRGINIA WOOLF 1938, 59

Unitary caring science invites us into an expanding universe and worldview that, if embraced, leads to a different song and contributes to a New Story for humanity and human caring. This New Story, coming from nursing and unitary thinking, is really an Old Story; it has been building across humanity for millions of years. In nursing, it has been building from Florence Nightingale onward but has been dwelling, often silently, behind the scenes of the dominant, outer world of material/physical/objective/hard Western science.

Unitary caring science as positioned here builds upon my original 1979 text, which began with a discussion of nursing as the Philosophy and Science of Caring; that discussion continued to evolve through other books, up to the 2nd edition in 2008 and beyond. (See appendix B for an overview of all other books, including those that are forthcoming).

This new work has evolved to a new level: *Unitary Caring Science: The Philosophy and Praxis of Nursing.* This book goes to another level of depth regarding a philosophy to inform and unify both science and practice/praxis. First is a clarification of the starting point of definitions, values, and worldview, allowing caring science to become more clearly seen as unitary caring science. This includes embracing metaphysics as well as embodied physical, empirical, concrete practice. It leads to a philosophically, ethically, and ontologically discipline-specific, informed unitary science paradigm to guide reverential sacred praxis for caring-healing and health.

If you seek to understand humans as a whole spiritual being, fully connected and evolving toward the Source with an infinite field of universal consciousness and Cosmic Love, and your starting point is the static physicality of Western metaphysics, R. D. Laing reminded us that "you cannot get there . . . it is like trying to make ice by boiling water" (Laing 1965, 24).

Disciplinary Definitions as Starting Point

Many of the problems of philosophy are of such broad relevance to human concerns, and so complex in their ramifications, that they are, in one form or another, perennially present. Though in the course of time, they yield in part to philosophical inquiry, *they may need to be rethought by each age in the light of . . . deepened ethical and [spiritual] experiences [and values]* (emphasis added).

ELIZABETH BEARDSLEY AND MONROE BEARDSLEY 1974, IX

Values Axiology

Axiology, or the study of values, serves as an important starting point for Unitary Caring Science, in that axiology is the philosophical study of value. By asking value questions of a human unitary science, which differs from conventional views of Western science, unitary caring science invites new questions about value as a starting point.

What is of worth? Examples include truth, beauty, aesthetics, dignity, honesty, integrity, love, caring, belonging, and humanity-planet-universe. Axiology is associated with the ethics of science and moral imperatives, those ultimate intrinsic values essential for preserving humanity and human caring. By introducing axiology as the starting point for science, we get to ask new questions of science as to where the moral values of caring, compassion, love, truth, beauty, unity of wholeness, and so on fit into a philosophy of science and, specifically, nursing as unitary caring science. We get to make explicit the issue of worth and address issues of what values are of

9

worth. Without a moral foundation to guide praxis of the discipline and to guide science, human caring can be threatened and humanity can be totalized and objectified, in danger of cruelty and non-caring scientific and clinical practices. This work introduces Veritas to convey nursing's morality and value commitment to timeless, enduring values that intersect with Caritas, which unites caring and love.

Exploration of axiology as the philosophical study of moral ideals, worth, commitment, ethics, and timeless values is a necessary foundation for unitary caring science. Any philosophy of science for nursing praxis depends upon notions of moral values, worth, and moral imperatives to sustain human caring, wholeness, dignity, and integrity of the human-universe–health-healing process.

Philosophy

A general orientation to philosophy is that it is an intense, reflective study of phenomena of interest regarding knowledge, systems of thought, and notions of being. In general, both philosophy and science are engaged in a search for truth. For example, *Veritas*, the Latin word for truth, is consistent with a search for knowing as part of philosophy's search for truth. The broad concept of Veritas Aequitas conveys a search for truth and justice. It is a motto that stands for personal honor and truth in actions and justice, regardless of the circumstance. At least three major branches of philosophy are relevant to unitary caring science and caring-healing practices/praxis: metaphysics, ethics, and epistemology. These in turn, consciously or unconsciously, guide our worldview of the human-cosmos existence of "being/belonging" with respect to unitary caring science praxis and transformative principles for guided policy actions/sacred activism.

Cosmology

Cosmology is the branch of metaphysics that addresses the nature of the universe (Watson, Smith, and Cowley 2018 in press). It addresses questions about the universe that are beyond the scope of science, yet it is subsumed under the branch of metaphysics that is beyond physics. Cosmology per se is beyond the focus of the philosophy of science addressed here, although cosmology is increasingly becoming a focus of concern regarding the universe itself and how it serves as the larger sacred context. Our collective story of the universe is allowing for either the infinite evolution of humanity or a totalizing of a human-planet universe.

Unitary caring science embraces a cosmology that honors the universe as context, consistent with Berry (1988). That is, the universe is the primary revelation of the Divine, the primary sacred source of existence, allowing the universe to be seen and experienced as joyous, filled with beauty, mysterious, wondrous, celebratory—a basic goodness of being and belonging together. The emerging cosmology is a response to the growing crisis of society and civilization in which the Old Story is no longer adequate for addressing the survival of the planet and humanity.

Metaphysics (summarized from various sources)

- **1a** is considered the first branch of philosophy, a division concerned with the fundamental nature of reality and being that includes ontology, cosmology, and often epistemology.
- **1b** ontology defines what it means "to be"; what is an existence worldview—for example, separatist versus unity.
- **1c** constitutes abstract philosophical studies, a study of what is outside objective experience, beyond the physical plane.
- **2** metaphysics describes what is beyond physics—the nature and origin of reality itself, the immortal soul, and the existence of a supreme being. Opinions about these metaphysical topics vary widely, since what is being discussed cannot be observed or measured or even truly known to exist. So, most metaphysical questions are still far from having a final answer.

In summary for our purposes here, metaphysics has two basic meanings (Watson, Smith, and Cowley 2018): (1) a branch of philosophy about one's worldview—for example, ontology of being; and (2) a branch of philosophy beyond the physical, inviting non-physical reality into our worldview and notions of being human. Metaphysics is especially relevant for exploring new explanatory unitary energy models of non-physical healing, beyond the body physical, and incorporating concepts such as non-local consciousness and new meta-paradigm concepts for spiritual healing, prayer, distant healing, and so on, for example.

Ontology

Ontology is the philosophical study of the nature of being, becoming, existence, or reality as well as constituting the basic categories of being and categories related to being, according to Merriam-Webster (https://www.merriam-webster.com/dictionary/metaphysics, accessed December 15, 2016). Traditionally listed as a part of the major branch of philosophy known as metaphysics, ontology often deals with questions concerning what entities exist or can be said to exist. Ontology as a philosophical enterprise is theoretical; it also has practical applications. Indeed, ontology and the nature of our unitary being inform and guide moral caring-healing practices, that is, praxis, whereby Caritas becomes a manifestation of discipline-specific unitary caring science praxis.

Ethics

What is the right thing to do when one is faced with two equally conflicting, untenable choices? The study of ethics and exploration of ethics in unitary caring science takes us back to axiology. The ethical dilemmas in nursing and medical care are tied to values and morality.

This rhetorical dilemma and quest for values and living values to which one ascribes becomes the basis for ethics and ethical decision-making. The notion of morality and values precedes ethics in that morality calls us to make the most morally correct value decision, for example, "the human should always be honored as an end in and of itself and not as a means to an end." This core value and moral imperative is in contrast to a clinical, professionally detached approach, which reduces the human to the moral status of an object whereby professionals can justify doing something to another person as object that they would not do to a whole person such as themselves. Therein, doing harm is theoretically justified because the decision was guided by a worldview and moral-ethical principles, which justify separation and distancing—a rule-driven, decision-making model. This approach is in contrast to a relational worldview of unity and complexity and connections, which transcend rules and principles, on behalf of human principles and a relational worldview that considers the whole versus the parts.

Ethics, which rely on objective rational decisions alone, often result in suffering and inhumane decisions that affect the lives of everyone involved. Parker Palmer has framed these objective ethical ways of knowing and what counts as evidence as a form of violence—thus, even our ways of knowing and what counts as knowledge have epistemological consequences and conditions. Epistemology, how we know what we know, becomes an ethic that affects our worldview, our human existence, our relationship with self/other/Mother Earth/, our universe (Palmer 2004).

Various theories and rule-driven principle-based models for ethical decision-making are prevalent in fields of biomedical ethics; examples include deontological ethics and utilitarian ethics, or rights-based models. However, these ethical positions are rule-driven and principle-guided, in contrast to unitary caring ethics of connection, relations, context, complexity, personal meaning. For example, instead of asking a simple question such as "in this situation, under these circumstances, do we follow principles, distancing, and rules," perhaps we may need to ask instead, *what is the kindest thing we can do* (inspired by Sarah Eagger, MD, United Kingdom).

Ethics of Unitary Caring Science

The counterpoint to conventional science and conventional approaches to bioethics is the worldwide work of Emmanuel Levinas (1969), who positioned the Ethics of Belonging as the starting point for all science, informing the Ontology of Being as one of belonging to Universal Cosmic Love. This Levinian ethic positions belonging against the separatist view, which disconnects humans from the life force energy of Universal Love. This ethic is tied back to axiology and values; what is truly valued and necessary to sustain moral imperatives?

Levinas (1969) noted that while he has been recognized for his ethical, moral, philosophical worldview, what was of most interest to him was the search for the holy. He acknowledged that all humans "belong" to the infinite field of Cosmic Universal Energy as the starting point, before the Ontology of Being.

Sidebar

Whereas Martin Heidegger (1927) focused on the Ontology of *Dasein*—being human and care as a way of being—Levinas declared that an Ethics of Belonging comes before the Ontology of Being. This introduces a higher level of unitary abstractions (in spite of Heidegger's notion of *Dasein* positing being human as special ways of being). Likewise, while Heidegger's view of being human and care is an ontological way of being in the world, Levinas posed belonging as a higher order, the ethical-philosophical starting point for science.

Levinas's ethical-moral foundation served as a foundation of caring science as Sacred Science (Watson 2005). Likewise, it serves as an ethical foundation for unitary caring science and metaphysics. I, too, am drawn to that which is holy, mysterious, mystical, and unknowable but fully known and experienced by all of humanity across time. Likewise, this perspective now intersects with unitary science and views of a quantum universe, uncovering and revealing the connectedness and oneness of all. We all reside in the universal cosmic field of energy.

Such a stance creates a clearing and open space to enter another horizon of being-belonging as one. That is, human-universe being-belonging moves beyond principles and objectives, the rationality of strict ego, the physical plane, and invites concepts such as energy, spirit, and universal consciousness into the discourse of science—indeed, invites the sacred into our science (Watson 2005). An evolved Ethics of Belonging allows for both the embodiment of unity of the whole person and the reality of immanence and transcendence as one whole.

Epistemology

Epistemology is the study of knowledge, the nature and process of knowledge. It also guides our ontological view of our relation to knowing, developing/creating/co-creating knowledge. Epistemology informs our consciousness about what counts as knowledge, how we know, and sources of knowing/knowledge.

An expanded epistemological perspective, a relational unitary caring science ontological worldview, is incorporated in critiquing knowledge and how we know what we know. We acknowledge multiple sources of knowledge and ways of knowing; for example, knowledge may come from rational, technical, empirical means. In Unitary Caring Science, however, we also embrace and honor intuitive, aesthetic, personal, spiritual, ethical sacred knowledge and "non-conventional knowing," non-scientific, metaphysical ways of knowing that do not conform to conventional medical science separatist worldviews.

Theories. Subsumed under epistemology are theories with various criteria in search of truth and knowledge. Unconsciously, our views of knowledge and ways of knowing affect what is credible, that is, our views of truth. Theories and philosophies of science are what frame disciplinary knowledge (Watson 2005, 12). Unitary caring science theories transcend but inform specific events; they seek explanations that reflect unitary ethical philosophical values for a field of study. Underlying any theory is a metaphysical-ontological context that can guide science and unitary caring science praxis.

Several dominant theories of truth are embedded in our culture.

Correspondence Theory of Truth. For example, one dominant view of truth is the correspondence theory of truth—that is, truth as objective, concrete, and physical. To be considered truthful, something has to correspond with reality data.

Coherence Theory of Truth. The coherence theory of truth has to show internal consistency within its context. It does not necessarily have to correspond to reality, but it must be coherent within its own paradigm.

Pragmatic Theory of Truth. Another view is the pragmatic theory of truth, which indicates that something is true if it is useful and workable for the purpose intended.

Unitary Caring Science Theory of Truth—*Aletheia* (Greek origin)

The theory of truth that both corresponds to and is coherent with unitary caring science views of truth is the Greek view of truth—the *Aletheia* Theory of Truth. This view is related to beauty, harmony, essence; it is tied to the subjective, inner life of being-belonging. The ontology of Unitary Being is tied to criteria as a source for truth. *In other words, truth is not knowledge per se; rather, it is an ontological question.* However, in Western science, truth has been interpreted as an epistemological issue. The notion of truth and what counts as truth and knowledge informs and imprints our methods as well as what is legitimate as methods, what counts as knowledge, and what is credible in terms of truth statements.

However, in positing that unitary caring science is consistent with Aletheia views, we are acknowledging that truth is not an epistemological question; rather, it is an ontological question. Heidegger brought renewed attention to this view of truth. It is tied to the essence of meaning and is related to being, whereby the subject determines truth. This is especially relevant because unitary caring science works from the inner subjective life world of the other in a dynamic flow. Unitary caring science seeks to work in a pattern of synchronicity within the other's energetic frame of reference. For example, if someone has experienced something, that is a truth for them; it is related to the meaning the phenomenon holds for them and their ways of being-belonging in the world. In an evolved unitary caring science worldview, which embraces the fullness of humanity for unitary caring science praxis, we acknowledge that there are many truths and no one truth.

My definition of theory is from the Greek word *Theoria*, which means "to see" and "to seek" in an intellectual, philosophical, ethical way. It does not consider theory to be just a body of substantiated facts.

SCIENCE (WESTERN MEDICAL)
Science is not the same in all paradigms in terms of [ethics,] ontology, epistemology, methodology [and praxis]. (Lather 2007, 164)

Gary Rolfe (2011) posited that "social and medical science paradigms adopted by the academic discipline of nursing are no longer fit for purposes in the 21st century" (Rolfe 2011, 60). Western medical science is defined by objective knowledge or a system of knowledge that covers general truths and laws predictably based on general laws. Knowledge is known through testing questions using the scientific method and through concern with the physical-outer world. In this form of knowledge and view of science, the emphasis is on objectivism, analytic and experimental knowledge, in which we distance ourselves from both the process and the knowledge itself, as well as from our ways of knowing and, indeed, what counts as knowledge and knowing.

As noted earlier (Hills and Watson 2011, 39–42), Parker Palmer also critiqued this view of science and knowledge as harmful to our experience and inner knowing. Perpetuating the myth of objectivism, experimentalism, and analytic criteria for their own sake alone can be a form of violence and an act of cruelty.

This epistemological awareness of the philosophy of science and meaningful knowledge is important to current nursing discourse related to science itself. For example, Rosemarie Parse (2015) raised the question, is it Nursing Science or is it the Science of Nursing? Within the context of a philosophy of science, this is an important question.

Within a Western epistemological worldview, the Science of Nursing can be viewed as funded research focused on disease-related conditions and diagnosis-focused care models, with knowledge of parts as a phenomenon of interest. This contrasts with Parse, who acknowledges that Nursing Science is "the unique body of knowledge embedded in the extant nursing frameworks and theories that continue to be developed through research and creative conceptualization" (2015, 101).

Barrett (2017) raised the continuing question, again, what is Nursing Science? Who knows and who cares? She highlighted the current funding priorities of the National Institute of Nursing Research (NINR), which focus on knowledge development in areas such as "omics, e-science, translation science, biobehavioral science, symptom science and team science" (Barrett 2017, 129). She argued that this focus on knowledge development "might obliterate nursing's discipline-specific phenomenon of concern: the human-universe-healing process" (Barrett 2017, 129).

Unitary caring science lifts conventional Western medical science and its view of epistemology, with its distancing objective being particulate disease phenomena and criteria, to another level. The Caring Ethic of Belonging combined with the disciplinary phenomena of nursing, unitary views of the human being, and a unitary worldview becomes the new standard and starting point for unitary caring science, beyond the myth of Western medical science as the be-all and end-all for how we view knowledge and the truth of our world.

Thus, a New Story of science and knowledge emerges under an epistemology of the unitary ethic of being-belonging, not just as data and information and knowledge per se. This unitary view of science is one of connecting knowledge, not separating it. This evolved Unitary Caring view of science allows for knowing and knowledge that leads to a unity of science and spirit, physical and non-physical, and metaphysical phenomena, inviting knowledge of creativity, immanence-transcendence, and human flourishing. This philosophy of unitary science unites us with knowing, discovering, and developing knowledge rather than distancing us from detached knowledge "out there." In unitary caring science, knowing and knowledge are constantly evolving—connecting the ethic and starting point of belonging to the universal field of Cosmic Love, which connects and unites everything in the universe. Finally, unitary caring science integrates the axiology of core values and the Ethic of Belonging as the source for its ontological-epistemological orientation to the phenomena of caring, consciousness, wholeness within a unitary field of human-universe—health and human well-being/becoming (Barrett 2017; Phillips 2017).

Native Science

In developing a New Story of science, perhaps we are seeing the need to consider the Old Story and enduring "science" of indigenous peoples. There is a uniting and common worldview across each tribe and nation, although each has specific ways of honoring the oneness of all. Consistent with a unitary view, the indigenous world is based on an assumption of oneness or wholeness in contrast to Western science, which is based on the ontological assumption of separation. The other distinction of so-called Native Science is that it is tied to values of learning to live in "harmony, non-exploitative, non-polluting ways of honoring their relationship with Mother Earth. Native Science has a sacred basis and its teachings are tied to love and sacred respect for nature; it is non-invasive, communally based" (Harmon 1991, 83–85).

This worldview and indigenous story of knowledge is related to circles and cycles in the search for truth about balance, harmony, and peace with all living relations. Further, all relationships have a moral content. This moral aspect of relationship is similar to the original meaning of praxis and the Ethic of Belonging within unitary caring science. The Greek meaning of praxis conveys a moral, committed disposition to all actions. Finally, Native Science views non-physical phenomenon to be as fully real as physical reality; dreams, myths, "talk story," visions, spirit are all alive, and both worlds exist as a place to live.

An example:

In the early 1980s I spent time with an aboriginal tribe in Western Australia. One of the elders of the tribe said to me: "The white man always follows the road that is ahead. In our world we have Dreamtime. We do not follow the road that is ahead, already paved—we throw the road out ahead and dream it up." This experience and example is a reminder that in a unitary world, everything in the physical world comes from the non-physical. So we indeed can visualize and dream up our reality; if you can dream it, so you can create it. In unitary caring science we get to embrace the full range of knowing and honoring our unitary being and belonging in harmony and right relations with nature and the universe. This Native Science cosmology blends with unitary caring science, inviting us to re-inspirit and re-enchant our relationship with nature, the known and unknown, and all living things.

Praxis

There are numerous definitions and interpretations of praxis. A Google search of praxis yielded 34.5 million definitions and meanings (accessed August 8, 2017). They begin with the Greek origin of Aristotle's use of the word—implying a theory, lesson, or skill that is enacted, embodied, or realized, personally experienced, including his varied meanings such as "good" praxis and "bad" praxis. They extend to Marxist political calls for praxis in social political action. Praxis definitions apply more commonly to educational systems and educational activism. For example, the Brazilian educator and activist Paolo Freire (1970) called for "conscientization," translated as "consciousness raising" and "critical consciousness" for emancipation. These definitions and meanings extend to spiritual praxis in fields such as Buddhism, Christian mysticism, and esoteric practices; these practices include meditation and transcendence. This spiritual meaning of praxis implies an opening up to the full depth of experience of divine, infinite love, transcendence. In the spiritual realm of praxis, one has to "fully taste life" free from dogma of the mind.

Medical Praxis

The medical, more scientific use of the meaning of praxis often refers to the simple, literal transfer of cognitive and psychomotor skills into practice, as well as a transfer of knowledge into action. Praxis often indicates action beyond theory or the opposite of theory. It is something practical—that is, practical praxis.

From Nursing Praxis to Unitary Caring Science Praxis

A Google search of "nursing praxis" yielded 559,000 results (accessed August 8, 2017). The results included praxis explored in terms of values, art, reflection, and synchrony of knowing/doing/being, to committed action, to knowledge and action, to practice distinguished from theory, to praxis as closing the theory-practice gap, to caring praxis as framework, to feminist praxis. Indeed, a New Zealand journal called *Nursing Praxis* publishes practice-oriented articles; this journal was influenced by New Zealand's Maori indigenous culture. Praxis includes various uses in nursing literature, books, and articles that highlight the importance of value-guided actions, art and artistry, and the act of care in the moment, integrating knowing/being/doing as one artful act. Still other meanings indicate that praxis is the discipline's worldview/meta-paradigm, combining knowledge, theory, science, education, and practice as a holistic entity. Praxis is seen as a seamless coming together of theory, moral foundation, research-inquiry, and practice.

Closer to my view is the notion of praxis not simply as reflective, knowledge-guided action but as embodying certain qualities. These unitary qualities are moral and ethical commitments to human caring, healing, health, and the universe. My orientation to praxis also implies a philosophical quest to search for truth, beauty, aesthetics, creativity, evolution of human consciousness, and movement toward a moral community of caring-healing and peace, which nursing has always represented.

In Aristotelian terms, nursing praxis, in particular from Florence Nightingale onward, has been guided by a moral disposition to act rightly, to serve the whole person, to honor and preserve the dignity and integrity of the whole person in his or her life-world field. In the Aristotelian praxis language there is "good praxis" (*eupraxis*) and "bad praxis" (*dyspraxis*). This line of Aristotelian thinking relates to the concept of caring literacy, beyond skill and knowledge for competent action, which alone can be devoid of the ethical moral worldview of belonging (Watson 2017). The praxis of unitary caring science has the potential to awaken nurses and other practitioners to a lack or an unconscious awareness of moral praxis disposition, which is dependent upon one's worldview and ethical starting point.

Unitary caring science (UCS) praxis, therefore, is informed moral practice, practice that is guided by one's unitary worldview, values, ethics, theory, and disciplinary knowledge. It can be considered *eupraxis*—good, morally informed, committed, authentic acts of caring literacy. UCS praxis becomes a human ontological artistry of being-becoming—transcending in the moment—through knowledgeable caring-healing values based on actions of goodness, truth, connectedness, opening to the infinity of Cosmic Love, expanded consciousness, intentionality; this moral praxis is held together by a commitment to sustain human-planet oneness—all guided by an underpinning of the Unity of Human Beings and an Ethic of Belonging as foundational.

If UCS and the Ethic of Belonging are informed consciousness as the first principle of science and UCS nursing praxis calls forth informed moral action in the world, then nursing praxis is situated and grounded in *eupraxis*, or good praxis. *Eupraxis* in Greek ethics means to act rightly. Here, this is translated to act rightly, informed by moral ideals and the theoretical unitary knowledge of human caring, healing, and health-universe. Exploring a unitary caring science praxis as *eupraxis* takes Caritas to Veritas, which uncovers more fully and clearly the values disposition of the discipline and practice of nursing—that is, to embody and embrace Veritas; to act with and honor goodness, truth, beauty, commitment, dignity, and nobility in service to humankind. Caritas and Veritas represent what nursing has stood for, which is what nursing represents across time. By exploring unitary caring science praxis, we bring light to a New Story that nursing has to offer to the world.

Indeed, unitary caring science *eupraxis* (moral component of praxis for goodness and truth) is revealed through both Caritas and Veritas—morally informed disciplinary actions in the world. Some of the so-called good praxis actions have been referred to as Caritas Literacy—*eupraxis*—implying a practitioner's moral disposition and consciousness to exhibit caring, love, and compassion for all of humanity. The counterpoint of *eupraxis* is Caritas Illiteracy—*dyspraxis* (Watson 2017). *Dyspraxis* practices are devoid of a caring consciousness or an informed intentionality to act in the practitioner's best judgment "to put patients in the best condition for healing," to draw upon a praxis blueprint from Florence Nightingale.

Praxis, with its many meanings and definitions, can be used as a backdrop to expand and improve nursing, allowing for the full range of concrete discipline-specific actions in the world: from critical evolutionary consciousness praxis to spiritual praxis. It opens nursing to the full range of experiences of touching the divine, the holy, the full expression of infinite cosmic love, the transcendent, miracles, mystery, and mysticism—all within the unitary field of life and humanity across the sacred circle of life-death-rebirth.

This range of praxis, from the concrete to the spiritual realm, parallels Marlaine Smith's findings (Smith 1999, 22–25), which unify Martha Rogers's science of unitary human beings (SUHB) with extant caring theories (Rogers 1994). One unitary area of caring science and SUHB is "caring is a way of experiencing the infinite"—that is, allowing for transcendence of the physical-material world, considered the highest form of knowing. Knowing includes Divine Love, ontological mystery, and spiritual union, thus expanding the limits of openness. So, just as praxis transcends multiple meanings, definitions, and levels of action in the world, so does unitary caring science praxis. Unitary caring science praxis can be considered *eupraxis*; it spans the entire horizon of being/doing/knowing/ becoming—from practical praxis to transpersonal-transcendent praxis.

Unitary caring science praxis has the potential to elevate the consciousness of individuals and all of humanity, since everyone resides within one unitary field. This perspective is noted by David Hawkins (2002), who posits and affirms that if any one person evolves in his or her consciousness, it contributes to the evolution of the consciousness of all of humanity. UCS praxis for nursing has an even greater moral imperative, going back to the Greek meaning of praxis as having a moral disposition and commitment to the betterment of humankind. *Eupraxis* of unitary caring science, with its moral-value foundation of Caritas and Veritas, is increasingly called for in our depersonalized, dehumanizing, institutional-corporate daily practices, whether these practices are experienced and witnessed in educational, political, economic, or medical systems.

Summary

Our starting point for science—knowledge and what counts as knowledge—informs and dictates where we end up. If our starting point for science and knowledge development is objectively value-neutral, without attention to moral imperatives for the human-universe, nursing is in danger of becoming extinct as a discipline. If value-neutral approaches are combined with an ontology of separation and objective parts on a material-rationalist plane of existence—the Era I–Paradigm I mind-set (particulate-deterministic phenomena) or even Era II–Paradigm II (interactive parts model)—then education, knowledge, and research would focus on generating more and more pieces of data that conform to Western empirical views of science, without clarity of the values or the ethical, philosophical, ontological, epistemological foundation that underpinned the starting point. Thus, they would offer no guide to inform and sustain human caring moral action/praxis.

All knowledge and what counts as knowledge is ultimately based on values, an ethic, a philosophy, an ontological worldview, and an epistemology of knowledge and what counts as knowledge. Western science views of knowledge per se do not advance knowledge of UCS; neither does a particulate paradigm for disciplinary knowledge advance nursing praxis. A unitary philosophy and moral-ethical value of belonging are needed to evolve to a new view of unitary caring that informs both the discipline of nursing and its praxis-*eupraxis*. Praxis-*eupraxis* proclaims that some actions are good for their own sake.

Finally, this chapter offered an overview of core components of a philosophy of science, which is often missing in graduate and undergraduate nursing studies. However, a background and questioning of the history and philosophy of science and all of its vicissitudes, which inform praxis, are necessary.

At this time in nursing's history and maturing, theories and disciplinary knowledge and informed moral praxis are threatened, as the profession is at a crossroads (Grace et al. 2016). Without an awakening to the fullness of the nursing phenomenon and its disciplinary history–philosophy of science context for informing its moral praxis, the discipline is in danger of extinction (Barrett 2017). Nursing itself, unless it evolves toward its finest *eupraxis*, can unknowingly contribute to the totalizing of humanity and *dyspraxia* in our world.

Reading List

Aristotle (2004). *The Nicomachean Ethics*. Trans. J.A.K. Thomson. London: Penguin.

Barrett, E. (2017). "Again, What Is Nursing Science?" *Nursing Science Quarterly* 30 (2): 129–33.

Bernstein, R. J. (1983). *Beyond Objectivism and Relativism: Science, Hermeneutics, and Praxis*. Oxford: Basil Blackwell.

Berry, T. (1988). *The Dream of the Earth*. Sacramento, CA: Sierra Club.

Carr, W., and S. Kemmis. (1986). *Becoming Critical: Education, Knowledge, and Action Research*. London: Falmer.

Chinn, P. L., and M. K. Kramer. (2008). *Integrated Theory and Knowledge Development in Nursing*. 7th edition. St. Louis, MO: Mosby.

Foucault, M. (1972). *The Archaeology of Knowledge*. London: Tavistock.

Foucault, M. (1977). *Power/Knowledge*. Ed. C. Gordon. New York: Pantheon.

Friere, P. (1972). *Pedagogy of the Oppressed*. New York: Penguin.

Gadamer, H.-G. (1976). *Philosophical Hermeneutics*. Berkeley: University of California Press.

Gadamer, H.-G. (1977). *The Relevance of the Beautiful*. Ed. R. Bernasconi. Cambridge: Cambridge University Press.

Gadamer, H.-G. (1979). *Truth and Method*. London: Sheed and Ward.

Harman, W. W. (1991). *A Re-examination of the Metaphysical Foundations of Modern Science*. Sausalito, CA: Institute of Noetic Sciences.

Harvey, A. (2009). *The Hope: A Guide to Sacred Activism*. Melbourne, AR: Institute for Sacred Activism.

Hawkins, D. R. (2002). *Power vs. Force*. Carlsbad, CA: Hay House.

Heidegger, M. (1977). *Basic Writings: From Being and Time to the Task of Thinking*. New York: Harper and Row.

Kuhn, T. (1970 [1962]). *The Structure of Scientific Revolutions*. 2nd edition. Chicago: University of Chicago Press.

Laing, R. D. (1965). *The Divided Self*. London: Pelican Book.

Lather, P. (2007). *Getting Lost: Feminist Efforts toward a Double(d) Science*. New York: State University of New York Press.

Lather, P. (2010). *Engaging Science*. New York: Peter Lang.

Levinas, E. (1969). *Totality versus Infinity*. Pittsburgh: Duquesne University Press.

Marx, K., and F. Engels. (1976). *The German Ideology*. Moscow: Progress Publishers.

Phillips, J. (2017). "New Rogerian Theoretical Thinking about Unitary Science." *Nursing Science Quarterly* 30 (3): 223–26.

Popper, K. R. (1965 [1962]). *Conjectures and Refutations: The Growth of Scientific Knowledge*. New York: Harper Torchbooks.

Reason, P. (1988). *Human Inquiry in Action*. London: Sage.

Reed, P. G., and N. B. Crawford Shearer. (2011). *Nursing Knowledge and Theory Innovation: Advancing the Science of Practice*. New York: Springer.

Rogers, M. E. (1970). *An Introduction to the Theoretical Basis of Nursing*. Philadelphia: F. A. Davis.

Rolfe, G. (2011). "Practitioner-Centered Research: Nursing Praxis and the Science of the Unique." In P. G. Reed and N. B. Crawford Shearer, eds.,

Nursing Knowledge and Theory Innovation: Advancing the Science of Practice. New York: Springer, 59–74.

Sarter, B. (1988). "Philosophical Sources of Nursing Theory." *Nursing Science Quarterly* 1 (2): 52–59.

Smith, M. K. (1999). "What Is Praxis?" In *Encyclopaedia of Informal Education.* Accessed August 8, 2017. http://infed.org/mobi-what-is-praxis/.

Teilhard de Chardin, P. (1955). *The Phenomenon of Man.* Toronto: R. P. Pryne.

Watson, J. (1999). *Postmodern Nursing and Beyond.* Edinburgh, Scotland: Churchill-Livingstone.

Watson, J. (2005). *Caring Science as Sacred Science.* Philadelphia: F. A. Davis.

Watson, J. (2008). *Nursing: The Philosophy and Science of Caring.* Revised ed. Boulder: University Press of Colorado.

Watson, J. (2012). *Human Caring Science.* Sudbury, MA: Jones and Bartlett.

Watson, J., M. Smith, and R. Cowley. (2018 in press). "Unitary Caring Science: Disciplinary Evolution of Nursing." In W. Rosa, S. Horton-Deutsch, and J. Watson, eds., *Handbook for Caring Science.* New York: Springer.

Woolf, V. (1938). *Three Guineas.* London: Hogarth.

Other websites:

https://www.merriam-webster.com/dictionary/praxis. Accessed August 8, 2017.

https://www.google.com/search/praxis. Accessed August 9, 2017.

https://www.google.com/search?client=safari&rls=en&q=nursing+praxis +definition. Accessed August 8, 2017.

Part Two

CHAPTER TWO

From Caring Science to Unitary Caring Science

The Maturing of the Discipline of Nursing

This chapter provides an overview of the evolution of Watson's caring science model and the Theory of Transpersonal Human Caring. It extends earlier discourse about the disciplinary foundation of nursing and the placement of caring within the meta-paradigm. This evolutionary intellectual discourse in the nursing literature is helping to reconcile previously disparate discourse and moves from Caring Science to Unitary Caring Science in harmony with the evolution of nursing's paradigmatic discourses.

Evolution Summary

This disciplinary turn offers a new synthesis for an evolved disciplinary consciousness. The result: (1) Unitary Caring Science for maturing the discipline; (2) an evolved Unitary Transformative view of nursing phenomena; (3) an affirming of Era III–Paradigm III thinking (unitary, ethic of belonging, non-physical, metaphysical, transcendent, and non-local consciousness phenomena as human experiences) as core to the discipline of nursing knowledge and theories; and (4) an evolved global consciousness toward a Quantum Unitary Universe for survival—that is, a cosmology of oneness of all, for human-planet survival.

Historical Context

In recent years, harmony and convergence have emerged between two historically parallel, non-intersecting developments in nursing: the science of Unitary Human Being (SUHB) (Martha Rogers) and caring science (CS) (Jean Watson). This contemporary convergence has evolved toward a unitary caring science worldview (Smith 1999, 2002, 2008; Watson and Smith 2008; Cowling, Smith, and Watson 2008). This contemporary mind-set of convergence has emerged from an ongoing critique of the original, dominant disciplinary meta-paradigm posed by Jacqueline Fawcett (1984): Person → Health → Environment → Nursing (which did not include caring in the foundational meta-paradigm underlying the discipline of nursing).

The generally accepted original disciplinary meta-paradigm, posed by Fawcett, about what constitutes core concepts of nursing has been challenged over the past several decades. Competing discourse from various scholars has identified at least three lingering philosophical and intellectual gaps, expanding the evolution of meta-paradigm thinking.

For example, seminal intellectual critique expanded the original discourse, raising new questions:

- The tautology of nursing as a concept located within the meta-paradigm (Conway 1985)
- Caring as a missing core concept in the meta-paradigm (Newman, Sime, and Corcoran-Perry 1991)
- Lack of clarity of philosophical paradigmatic assumptions related to the disciplinary concepts identifying the three major paradigms that guide nursing science and research:

o   Particulate-Deterministic (P-D)

o   Interactive-Integrative (I-I)

o   Unitary Transformative (UT) (Newman et al. 2008).

Newman and colleagues (2008) continued to critique the disciplinary assumptions in "The Focus of the Discipline Revisited."
This publication moved the disciplinary discourse regarding the
meta-paradigm to another level in two important ways:

1. The authors offered an explicit unifying defining statement of
    nursing by designating "Nursing as Caring" in the human health
    experience, making a case for including caring in the meta-
    paradigm (Newman et al. 2008, 16).

2. Further, this seminal publication critiqued and expanded how
    understanding is enhanced in relation to the paradigmatic and
    philosophical lens with which phenomena are viewed:

    o   Particulate-Deterministic (P-D)— literal, objective, concrete
        view; empirics, quantitative rational-cognitive knowing

    o   Interactive-Integrative (I-I)—qualitative, aesthetic, ethical
        metaphorical meaning interpretation

    o   Unitary Transformative (UT)—unitary, evocative,
        transcendent-spiritual level, experience of infinity, Divine
        Love, bliss.

By critiquing the different paradigmatic levels, one can identify
a dialectical intellectual gap. That is, by reasserting what has been
widely held since Florence Nightingale, nursing practice becomes
a unified whole. Therefore, the first two levels of paradigm thinking—P-D and I-I—are part-focused, inconsistent with the unified
whole thinking of UT as the more highly evolved consciousness
level.

Further, these scholars posited that the discipline cannot fully
mature until the meta-paradigm concepts are located within the
evolved philosophical lens of UT. This position asserted, the first
two paradigms restrict nursing phenomena and limit nursing

knowledge since they are located within a parts model, inconsistent with a whole person unitary transformative worldview.

These nursing scholars further provided clarity and direction by offering a unifying concept of "Nursing as Caring and the human health experience" (Newman et al. 2008). By locating the definition within the UT paradigm, the concepts and definition of Nursing as Caring and the human health experience can now be viewed as a unified whole within that paradigm.

This development has emerged from a disciplinary critique regarding both the inclusion of caring in the meta-paradigm (Newman et al. 2008) and the location of nursing phenomena in their most mature paradigm, that is, evolving from Era I to Era III thinking—a unitary quantum worldview (Watson 1999, 2011). This evolution is consistent with UT paradigm thinking. For example, it moves from

- Era I—Particulate-Deterministic (P-C) to
- Era II—Interactive-Integrative (I-I) to
- Era III—Unitary Transformative (UT) as the most mature paradigm to accommodate nursing's human phenomena of wholeness, caring, health, presence, pattern, consciousness, energy, meaning, and so on (Newman et al. 2008).

Through the contemporary disciplinary discourse (Conway 1985; Newman, Sime, and Corcoran-Perry 1991; Newman et al. 2008; Smith 1999; Watson and Smith 2002; Cowling, Smith, and Watson 2008; Watson, Smith, and Cowling 2018 in press), the Caring in Nursing meta-paradigm has been established. Likewise, the Unitary Transformative paradigm and Era III thinking is now acknowledged as the most evolved mind-set, from Nightingale to current times, to address and embrace nursing's human phenomenon of wholeness.

However, these different paradigms can be resolved. A part-concept viewed at the P-D or I-I paradigm level can still be integrated into a UT unified whole person approach because UT accommodates all that is included before it. For example, one can have UT consciousness of the whole while attending to the part.

The metaphor of a hologram serves to clarify the point—for example, the whole is in the part and the part is in the whole. For example, the whole of caring consciousness resides in a single caring moment (Watson 1999, 2008, 2012).

Other Emerging Unitary Caring Science Theories

As part of the evolution of nursing theory and disciplinary scholarship, a series of nursing theories and seminal manuscripts can be identified as specifically contributing to the evolution of Unitary Caring Science and the converging of unitary themes. They include Rogers (1970); Newman (1994); Watson (2002, 2008, 2012); Parse (2014); Smith (1999); Watson and Smith (2002); Cowling, Smith, and Watson (2008).

As far back as 1987 (influenced by Smith, personal communication, 2017), Barbara Sarter (1988) examined the philosophical/theoretical systems underpinning Rogers's science of Unitary Human Being (SUHB), Rosemarie Parse's Theory of Human Becoming, Margaret Newman's Theory of Expanding Consciousness, and Watson's Transpersonal Caring Science. At the conclusion of her analysis, she identified five themes that constitute the development of a shared distinctive worldview: (1) an evolutionary process that portends constant change and transcendence, (2) health as evolution or transcendence, (3) open systems, (4) non-linear space-time, and (5) pattern. Sarter concluded, "These themes together form a potentially powerful . . . metaphysical and epistemological foundation for the further development of a variety of nursing theories" (Sarter 1987, 58). "She [Sarter] implied an emergent science with the potential for a coherent worldview from which other theories might merge . . . a Unitary Caring Science" (Watson, Smith, and Cowling 2018 in press).

These unitary themes and the ethic of belonging coincide with a current futuristic awareness of quantum physics principles and the intersection of these ideas with complexity science and chaos science. The evolution of an awakening consciousness of oneness is prominent in unitary caring science.

The cosmology of the unitary worldview is one of interconnectedness and undivided wholeness. Unitary refers to the view that humans and the environment are irreducible and integral. This is based on the assumption of a universe composed on contiguous, interpenetrating energy fields. Rogers (1992) states, "The energy field is the fundamental unit of the living and non-living" (p. 29). The universe consists of indivisible fields within fields, all vibrating. These energy fields have no boundaries; by their nature they are open, flowing, and continuously changing. Without boundaries and extending to infinity, fields are interconnected. This means that everything in the universe is interconnected; it is one whole. Each unit as well is coextensive with the entire universe (Rogers 1992). The universe is composed of "open energy systems constantly interacting and evolving with each other" (Newman 1994). This cosmology is supported by the ideas in both quantum physics and Eastern philosophies (Watson, Smith, and Cowling 2018 in press).

The most recent views of the convergence of unitary views of science within the metaphysical philosophy of science context are summarized by John Phillips (2017) in his description of emerging scientific knowledge, which he labels "selected views of science" (223 [reprinted with permission]):

- Everything manifests wave frequencies, vibrations, resonances of patterns and fields.
- The human body manifests wave frequencies and diversity.
- Spirit and soul are of the universe and are integral.
- Time and space do not exist in a unitary, integral universe.
- The universe manifests consciousness/awareness.
- The universe manifests thought, information, and knowledge.
- The universe has a process of communication, and communication can be non-local.
- Humans have a mind that is not confined to the brain.
- Humans are holoids of a holographic universe.

Discipline Informs the Profession

As noted, nursing has been evolving over the past four to five decades to clarify and articulate its disciplinary foundation. It is a sign of maturity for nursing to continue to seek relationships and commonalities of knowledge that influence the scope of its disciplinary foundation. Nursing continues to question and revise its theories and body of knowledge as part of its disciplinary maturity and self-reflection.

Caring Science—Philosophical Ethical Foundation of the Unitary Transformative Paradigm

Just as nursing has a responsibility to continue to question, revise, and mature within its disciplinary structure, nursing has a responsibility to continue to evolve its moral-ethical value covenant with humanity (Donaldson and Crowley 1978; Watson 2005).

While the nursing paradigm discourse has evolved and perhaps crystalized at the UT level, the ethical-moral foundation of nursing science continues to evolve. For example, the first ANS issue on ethics was published in 1979, and yet ethical nursing issues and concerns remain. Peggy Chinn's 2001 ANS editorial "Nursing and Ethics: The Maturing of a Discipline" highlighted the fact that ethical issues in nursing remain a major concern among nursing scholars and practitioners. Indeed, she acknowledged that the crisis in nursing and healthcare continues, and ethical issues guide how and if we survive as a discipline. She further advised that all nurse scholars need to be well versed in ethics and philosophy to address and analyze the serious issues we face.

Unifying Theories and Paradigms

As the evolved disciplinary discourse placed human caring within the UT paradigm, it invited a new conversation for an evolved view of an ethical-moral theoretical foundation of nursing and science. Theories and philosophies of science frame disciplinary knowledge; they transcend specific events and seek to provide universal explanations that can reflect the ethical-philosophical foundation and values for the entire field of study (Reed, Shearer, and Nicholl 2003, 12). Likewise, theories contain underlying ontological-philosophical-ethical assumptions about knowledge and values for humanity, human caring, health experiences, the environment, and science. Diverse theories (for example, of caring) and diverse paradigms of science (for example, Paradigm P-D, I-I versus UT) can unite or divide.

To broaden and expand the continual, evolving disciplinary debate, Watson and Smith (2002) critiqued these two dominant discourses to detect any commonalities or divergences between hidden ethical-ontological assumptions and paradigms—specifically, between caring science (CS) and its intersection with SUHB— that have emerged in contemporary nursing literature. In this work, foundational issues of CS and Watson's theory of Transpersonal Caring Science (TCS) and Rogers's SUHB uncovered a distinct unitary view of humans with a relational caring ontology and ethic that informs nursing as well as other sciences. The result was a trans-theoretical, trans-disciplinary view for nursing knowledge development: "This trans-theoretical position moved nursing toward theoretical integration and creative synthesis versus separation, away from the 'Balkanization' of different theories [and paradigms])" (Watson and Smith 2002, 452).

The result of this analysis and convergence was a unitary caring science that evokes both science and spirit. The further conclusion of this work was that it is possible for the discipline of nursing to maintain integrity of different theories and paradigms while facilitating and inviting a new discourse for nursing science: that is, one of seeking new creative and philosophical-ethical connections among emerging nursing developments.

With respect to paradigms of caring and holistic views, Smith (1999) explored another area: diverse, multiple theories of caring from the ontological-ethical level to detect if caring knowledge could be located within a UT holistic context that honored the unitary human. This seminal work uncovered five constitutive meanings of caring from a wide range of caring theories in nursing that affirmed congruence between caring knowledge and UT holistic thinking.

The results include the following ethical and relational ontological findings, consistent with UT and holistic thinking. These foundational elements have recently been positioned within the most current level of unitary caring science (Smith 1999, 22–25).

- **Unitary Caring is manifesting intention**—What we hold in our heart matters (Cowling, Smith, and Watson 2008). Everything is energy. Our pattern of consciousness, manifested through our feelings, thoughts, perceptions, attitudes, and values, co-creates the evolving, dynamic patterning of the environment . . . Intentions are non-local because of the interconnectedness of all. Caring is being aware of holding intentions for well-being, healing, peace; for enfolding loving-kindness and compassion in our hearts; and in trusting that through the quality of this intentional engagement, we are participating meaningfully in healing and well-becoming (Smith 1999, 2010, 2015; Phillips 2017).
- **Unitary Caring is appreciating pattern**—This concept was appropriated directly from Richard Cowling's (1999, 2000) work. He differentiated the process of appreciating from assessing. Appreciating is apprehending the beauty and complexity of human wholeness with gratitude and awe. In contrast to a stance of identifying problems or making judgments, caring is entering into a relationship with the curiosity to come to know the uniqueness of the other (person, family, or community), affirming the humanity/divinity revealed in relationship, and seeing the other as whole and complete in the moment (Smith 1999, 2010, 2015).
- **Unitary Caring is attuning to dynamic flow**—This refers to the process of rhythmic relating that occurs in the caring relationship. There is a sensing of where to place focus and

emphasis, what to say, how to move in-the-between. This sensing of vibration is amplified by finely tuning the heart in connection with the other. It is a phenomenon of resonance, or vibrating in synchrony. Caring is the ability to move in concert with the evolving patterning of healing and well-becoming (Phillips 2017; Smith 1999, 2010, 2015).

- **Unitary Caring is experiencing the Infinite**—In the intimate caring relationship there is a perception of transcendence of the physical and material world and an expansion of time and space. There is an expanded sense of self, including transcendent awareness. Higher consciousness and evolved patterns of knowing are potentiated. Living caring is surrendering to the enfolding and unfolding mystery of spiritual connectedness and divine love (Smith 1999, 2010, 2015).

- **Unitary Caring is inviting creative emergence**—Healing is a dynamic process of transformation involving change and growth. Unitary caring is nurturing that growth through exploring and supporting the person's chosen journey; helping the other to articulate what matters most in the moment, identifying strengths and obstacles to change, and mobilizing internal and external resources to support healing and well-becoming (Phillips 2017). It is bearing witness to suffering and holding space for this transformation to evolve. In unitary caring there is no prescribed outcome; instead, there is a process of guiding, sojourning with, and tending the birth of healing and well-becoming (Phillips 2017; Smith 1999, 2010, 2015). (Watson, Smith, and Cowling 2018 in press).

As nursing continues to advance and mature with clarity of its disciplinary foundation and these converging caring literacies, it affirms experiences such as "experiencing the infinite," thereby inviting a deeper philosophical ethic and evolving worldview. This caring science as sacred science (Watson 2006) affirms that the French philosopher Emmanuel Levinas's (1969) explication of the Ethic of

Belonging to the infinity of Universal Love comes before the ontology of separation (Watson 2005). Levinas's infinity of Universal Love expands and converges with Smith's concept of caring as experiencing the infinite and inviting creative emergence.

This perspective also affirms the full meaning of unitary caring science praxis, which allows science and spirit to merge, inviting infinity, transcendence, and evolving consciousness into the disciplinary discourse of moral praxis. Unitary caring science praxis is guided by the moral-ethical meaning of praxis, as committed, morally informed action. This meta-theoretical analysis expanded caring knowledge, deepening the ethical-moral underpinnings and meaning of unitary caring within the context of UT science, but it also united diverse theories of caring.

Watson's Theoretical Prelude to Unitary Caring Science

Earlier works on Caring Science (Watson 2005, 2008, 2012) were preliminary underpinnings of unitary caring science. For example, the following tenets and assumptions identify the sacred nature of Caring Science. They unite science and spirit, physical and metaphysical, immanent and transcendent. Further, these principles of transpersonal and sacred science include premises congruent with Phillips's (2017) current tenets of unity.

- Ethic of Belonging (to the infinity of universal cosmic love) as the first principle of science.
- Infinity of the human spirit.
- The ancient and contemporary cosmology of unitary, non-local consciousness—universal connection of all.
- Consciousness transcends time, space, and physicality, becoming part of the complex energetic pattern of one's life.
- A transpersonal caring moment becomes the "eternal now" in that the moment patterns the energetic field of synchrony, becoming part of the infinite complex pattern of life.

- A transpersonal caring moment can be a transformative turning point for healing.
- Caring and love are the most universal, tremendous, and mysterious of the cosmic forces; they comprise the primal and universal psychic energy.
- Love is the greatest source of all healing.
- Caring and love are critical to an evolving humanity and survival as a human civilization and a planet.
- Professional unitary caring praxis draws upon energetic caring-healing modalities and the ten Caritas Processes.

Affirmatives in Disciplinary Unitary Caring Science Evolution

The disciplinary developments and scholarly discourses have brought us to a mature meta-paradigmatic ground. These developments include:

- Defining "nursing as *caring* in the human health experience" (Newman et al. 2008, 4).
- Uncovering commonalities among diverse theories of caring when viewed from the perspective of ontological-ethical values converging with holistic UT paradigm views, affirming that caring is ultimately a relational ontology of wholeness and connections and a way of being-in-relation that shows up as:
   o A way of manifesting intentions, appreciating patterns, attuning to dynamic flow, experiencing the infinite; a way of inviting creative emergence (Smith 2002).
- Clarifying and identifying intersections between TCS and Rogers's SUHB within a Unitary Transformative paradigm— positing Unitary Caring Science as uniting energy-science and spirit.
- Another unique disciplinary discourse posed by Cowling, Smith, and Watson (2008) expanded the discussion by positioning three critical concepts distinct to nursing: wholeness, conscious-

ness, and caring. From this ethical and intellectual synthesis of disciplinary dialogue, the authors posed the term *ontological caring literacy* as a unitary caring science praxis to help affirm and sustain humanity, caring, and wholeness in our daily work and the world (Cowling, Smith, and Watson 2008, E41).

You can visit watsoncaringscience.org to view a video of my keynote speech at the Unitary Caring Science–2016 Boston Conference, the first joint conference of the IAHC-SRS (International Association of Human Caring and the Society of Rogerian Scholars).

CHAPTER THREE

Background

*Caritas and Theory of Transpersonal Caring**

Within the Unitary Transformative paradigm, everything is connected at the energetic, quantum level, and small acts have a ripple effect in the field. Human beings are viewed as whole. Caring moments within the Unitary Transformative paradigm have been perceived as a "mutuality" of human-to-human patterning (Newman 1991). Watson refers to these human caring moments as transpersonal moments, whereby a caring moment transcends time, space, and physical presence (Watson 1999, 2005) and creates a new field of possibilities (Watson, Porter O'Grady et al. 2018 in press, used with permission).

Caritas comes from the Latin word meaning to cherish, to appreciate, and to give special, if not loving, attention to. It represents charity and compassion, generosity of spirit. It connotes something very fine, indeed, something precious that needs to be cultivated and sustained (Watson 2008, 39).

---

* Parts of this chapter are extracted and modified from Watson 2008, 39–43, and from a pending publication by Watson, Porter O'Grady, and colleagues 2018 in press.

Caritas is closely related to the word *Carative* from my original (1979) text on caring science. However, now, using the terms *Caritas* and *Veritas*, I intentionally invoke Love, which makes explicit the connection between caring and Love, Love in its fullest universal infinite sense, developed in the philosophy of Emmanuel Levinas (1969) and explored in my 2005 text, *Caring Science as Sacred Science.*

I shifted the language of caring from Carative to Caritas after I had an accident and went through an inner contemplative healing journey of my own. After my "down time" (see Watson 2005 for more background of that experience) and once I re-engaged in my own scholarship, I realized that the terms *Carative* and *factors* were too constraining and dense for the flowing I wanted to convey. Also, I wanted to give caring a deeper, more ethical, human-to-human meaning. So for several reasons, the word Caritas evokes and communicates a meaning I wished to convey, of beauty and heart-to-heart, authentic philosophical connections. The word Caritas brought caring and Love together in a way Carative did not.

Bringing caring and Love together more clearly places nursing within the Unitary Transformative paradigm but affirms the ethic of oneness, of belonging to the Infinite field of Universal Cosmic Love. The ten Caritas Processes have now been affirmed as universals, validated from diverse cultures around the world.

Caritas, uniting Love and caring, makes more explicit unitary of oneness connections among caring, Love, and healing. This process creates an opening/alignment with source (Infinite Love) as the greatest source of all healing—inner and outer healing for self and others. And healing and wholeness can be understood as one-being-in-right-relation-with the source (open to the Infinite).

While health may be considered to represent expanding consciousness, Love is the highest level of consciousness and the greatest source of all healing in the world. This connection with Love as a source for healing extends from the individual self to nature and the larger universe, which is evolving and unfolding. This cosmology and worldview of caring and Love—Caritas—is both grounded and metaphysical; it is immanent and transcendent with the co-evolving human in the universe.

When we include and bring together caring and Love in our work and our lives, we discover and affirm that nursing, like teaching, is more than a job. It is a life-giving and life-receiving career for a lifetime of growth and learning. It is maturing in an awakening and an awareness that nursing has much more to offer humankind than simply an extension of an outdated model of medicine and medical–techno-cure science. Nursing helps sustain human dignity and humanity itself while contributing to the evolution of human consciousness, helping to move toward a more humane and caring moral community and civilization (Watson 2008, 40). We move from Caritas to Communitas.

Further, we are asked to reconnect nursing's disciplinary source to its noble moral Veritas Eupraxis Praxis heritage and history to cultivate a new awareness/affirmation of the morals, values, and virtues of nursing, both ancient and emerging, needed for a new worldview—a cosmology that invites and welcomes the energy of universal virtues, values of caring and Love, back into our lives and our world. Such thinking calls forth a sense of reverence and sacredness with regard to our work, our lives, and all living things. It incorporates art, science, and spirituality as they are redefined.

As we enter into a maturing of unitary caring science and an evolved Caritas–Veritas Praxis–(Eupraxis) Literacy as a professional, discipline-specific theoretical map, we are simultaneously challenged to relocate ourselves in these emerging moral ideals and ideas and question for ourselves how this work speaks to us as a discipline and a practice profession. Each person is asked, invited, if not enticed, to examine, explore, challenge, and question for him- or herself and for the discipline the critical intersections between the personal and the professional. In this awakening of the unitary field, the personal *is* the professional. We practice who we are, we teach who we are, we live who we are as a person—thus, this work requires a personal transformation for our own journey to a higher level of consciousness. We can still witness a range of nursing and nurse's practice; however, a unitary Caritas-Veritas–conscious nurse, a unitary Caritas-Veritas–conscious practitioner, continues the journey throughout his or her life career as a living Caritas-Veritas journey, constantly seeking new levels of personal spiritual growth and moral consciousness evolution—moving ever closer to Teilhard de Chardin's Omega point or seeking to reach ever more to touch Levinas's infinite field of Cosmic Universal Love.

At a global level, we witness an evolution of human consciousness around the world among nurses and the general public, seeking spiritual dimensions of life and new meanings when faced with physical-health crises. In many ways the public is more evolved in what it wants for health and healing than US Westernized hospital cultures of medical treatment as the be-all and end-all.

This work calls each of us into our deepest self to give new meaning to our lives and work, to explore how our unique gifts, talents, and skills can be translated into compassionate human caring–healing service for self and others and even the planet earth. We honor the wounded healer within, so the wounds we carry and for which we seek healing become lessons for humility—opening our hearts to have more and more compassion instead of shutting down our hearts. To heal self, we face the shadow-light dance of our own life journey. We celebrate our hurts as lessons without apologies, giving us more strength, confidence, and courage to be Caritas.

It is hoped that at some level this work will help all of us in the caring-healing professions to remember who we are and why we have come here to do this work in the world.

VALUE ASSUMPTIONS OF CARITAS

- Caring and Love are the most universal, tremendous, and mysterious cosmic forces; they comprise the primal and universal source of energy.
- Often this wisdom is overlooked or we forget, even though we know people need each other in loving and caring ways.

- If our humanity is to survive and if we are to evolve toward a more loving, caring, deeply human and humane moral community and civilization, we must sustain Love and caring in our lives, our work, our world.

- Since nursing is a caring profession, its ability to sustain its caring moral ideals, ethics, and philosophy for professional practices will affect the human development of civilization and nursing's mission in society.

- As a beginning, we have to learn how to offer caring, Love, forgiveness, compassion, and mercy to ourselves before we can offer authentic caring and Love to others.

- We have to treat ourselves with loving-kindness and equanimity, gentleness and dignity before we can accept, respect, and care for others within a professional caring-healing model.

- Nursing has always held a caring stance with respect to others and their health-illness concerns.

- Knowledgeable, morally informed, ethical caring is the essence of Caritas-Veritas consciousness for professional nursing values, commitments, and competent-literate actions; it is the most central and unifying source to sustain its covenant with society and ensure its survival.

- Preservation and advancement of unitary caring science values, knowledge, theories, philosophies, morality, ethics, and critical Caritas-Veritas literacy practices are ontological, epistemological, and clinical endeavors; these endeavors are the source and foundation for sustaining and advancing the discipline and the profession.

(ADAPTED FROM WATSON 1985, 32, 2008, 41)

When love moves through us it inspires all we do . . .
Love and compassion must begin with kindness toward ourselves . . .
One of the greatest blocks to loving kindness is our own sense of unworthiness.

KORNFIELD (2002, 95, 101, 100)

Caring is underpinned and motivated by our humanistic-altruistic values system. This inner calling continues to lay the foundation for the moral ideals and Caritas-Veritas Literacy underlying caring science/unitary caring science—it is here in this value system that we honor the unity of our shared humanity. By affirming the oneness of being-belonging, awakening to the reality that what we do to others we do to ourselves, and working from a moral Veritas value system of caring and Love, we live joy.

> I slept and dreamed
> That life was joy.
> I awoke and saw that life was service.
> I acted and behold service was joy.
>
> TAGORE

As a given, caring must be grounded within a set of universal human values—kindness, concern, and Love of self and others. As one matures into a disciplinary grounded professional model of caring-healing and health in its broadest and deepest dimensions, one must cultivate an awareness and intentionality to sustain such a guiding vision for one's life and work. Caritas in its original and evolved sense honors the gift of being able to give and receive with a capacity to love and appreciate all of life's diversity and its individuality within each person.

Such a system helps us tolerate difference and view others through their subjective worldview rather than through ours alone. It is in this living, evolving Caritas-Veritas consciousness that we celebrate diversity while also awakening to the oneness of the human-life-universe.

Regardless of whether one is conscious of one's own philosophy and moral value system, it is affecting the encounters, relationships, and moments we have with our self and others. These humanistic-altruistic values can be considered our truths, our moral integrity to offer compassionate human caring in service to our world.

These emotions of Love, kindness, gentleness, compassion, equanimity, and so on are intrinsic to all humans. These emotions and experiences are the essence of what makes us human and what deepens our humanity and our connection with spirit, the Divine. This awareness is what connects us with the source from which we draw our sacred breath for life itself. It is here where we access our energy and creativity for living and being; it is here, in this model, that we yield to the transpersonal, honoring a unity with all. Awakening to this reality of oneness and surrendering our individual ego-self reminds us that we belong to the universe of humanity and all living things.

We are now called, invited, and challenged to take our moral values and our consciousness to a deeper level in our maturity, our awareness, our experiences and expressions—leading to informed moral Caritas-Veritas Literacy. This is a path of deepening our consciousness of who and what we are that prepares us for a lifelong journey of purpose and meaning and an inner calling for fulfilling this precious life world.

The Theory of Transpersonal Caring

The Theory of Transpersonal Caring (Watson 1985, 1988, 1999, 2008, 2012, 2017) has continued to evolve since the mid-1980s. It likewise acknowledges caring as a serious epistemic, ontological phenomenon that now makes explicit the fact that transpersonal is located within the field of unitary caring science. It is guided by the underlying ethic and worldview of unity of consciousness; transpersonal caring acknowledges Love as the highest level of consciousness and the source of all healing. Further, this early work resulted in caring becoming the basic ontology of being/belonging within the Era III context of non-local consciousness phenomena (Watson 1999, 2011). The term *transpersonal* refers to a "dynamic, energetic spirit manifesting aspects of being and becoming in the caring moment." Transpersonal also means "beyond the ego," whereby one is authentically present in the moment, connecting with and open to the infinite field of possibility (Watson 2002a, 12, 2002b).

Transpersonal caring is life-giving and life-receiving, making the connection between caring/Caritas and Love, allowing for an evolution of consciousness. Caritas Consciousness and a "caring moment" are transpersonal, beyond the ego of either; they constitute an *eternal now*. An "eternal now" unites past, present, and future in the "now moment." The concept of the "eternal now," of "transpersonal caring moment," evolved from Alfred North Whitehead's process philosophy and process metaphysics (Whitehead 1925, 1978). The study of Whitehead's philosophy influenced my development of the transpersonal caring moment and the concept of the eternal now (Watson 1985, 1988).

Transpersonal human caring moments and connections include the nurse's consciousness, intentionality, and unique authenticity, combined with energetic healing presence and actions, through full use of self through movements, senses, touch, sounds, words, colors, and forms in which he or she transmits and reflects the person's condition back to that person . . . The Transpersonal caring moment can be transcendent in that it opens up shared access to a spirit-filled source of infinity. Such (transpersonal) caring connections in turn help to restore inner harmony, while also contributing to the patient and nurse finding meaning in the experience. However, the origin of the meaning for both resides within, rather than existing without, outside. In this process the nurse is attending to . . . preserving the dignity of the person . . . as an important end in and of itself. (Watson 2012, 70–71)

Connecting with the subjective world of self/other has the potential to "touch the higher spiritual sense of self or the soul. As such, transpersonal human caring occurs as an I-Thou Relationship. It helps the person gain a sense of inner harmony. This process has the potential to generate a self-healing process . . . A [transpersonal] caring moment becomes part of the life history of each person. Transpersonal moments transcend time, space, and physicality; each moment informs the next moment, affecting the life field of each person. All we have in life are moments. A [transpersonal] moment is a moral-philosophical ideal of informed conscious intentional action" (Watson 2012, 71). It is not an interpersonal technique—rather, it is a moral-ethical authentic presence of being/becoming in the moment, to preserve the protection, enhancement, and preservation of humanity and human dignity:

> Transpersonal Caring is transcendent, in that it allows the presence of the geist or spirit; the moment is an "eternal-now" [that] expands the limits of openness and has the ability to expand human capacities for healing. A transpersonal moment potentiates a new human-environment field patterning, opening to the human dynamic expressions of love . . .
>
> Such an ideal of intersubjectivity and spirit-to-spirit connection is grounded in a belief that "we learn from one another how to be human by identifying ourselves with others, finding our dilemma in our self." For example[,] any one person's story could be anyone's story. What we all learn from these moments is self-knowledge. The self we learn about or discover is every self. It is universal—the human self. We learn to recognize ourselves in others. The comparison shows us what we are, what humanness is in general and in particular . . . it keeps alive our common humanity. This consciousness of transpersonal moments and connections helps us to morally avoid reducing our self and others to the moral status of object, whereby our own and another's humanity is totalized. (Watson 2012, 72)

In my theory of and original scholarship on caring science, I purposely use Caritas to indicate caring as more than a slogan, beyond the trivial meaning as a commodity to be marketed and sold and used in an exploitative way by systems and corporate thinking. Caritas moves caring beyond just "being nice," therefore dismissed as anything of substance. Quite the contrary: Caritas—combined now with Veritas morality—conveys a deep ethical, epistemic value foundation. Caritas brings the philosophy and ontology of oneness, wholeness, unity, and connection; it invites Cosmic Love and the universal field of Infinity into our daily life world. Unitary caring science ushers in an evolved model of science.

Within this evolved worldview, Caritas-Veritas Consciousness becomes a form of human literacy so greatly needed at this time in human history. This consciousness can happen in a flash, in a given moment, manifesting an energetic field of higher vibratory frequency because it holds energy of caring and Love. Margaret Newman (1994) posited "Health as Expanding Consciousness"; therefore, we may ask, what is the highest level of consciousness? It is Love or what Teilhard de Chardin labeled "the Omega point," meaning close to the Godhead, what Levinas identified as the Infinity of Universal Cosmic Love.

In my book *Postmodern Nursing and Beyond* (1999 [republished by Elsevier in 2011]), I call upon Gary Zukav's view of consciousness, connecting consciousness with energy and light (2013 [1979]). For example, if our intentional consciousness is to hold thoughts that are caring, loving, open, kind, and receptive, in contrast to attempts to control, manipulate, and exercise power, the consequences of our actions will be significantly different. The consequences are based on different levels of consciousness.

Emotions such as anger, jealousy, fear, and hatred are low-frequency energy, which lowers the frequency of one's light. Emotions such as Love, compassion, caring, kindness, and forgiving raise the frequency of one's being. When one's consciousness shifts, the person's experience shifts (Watson 1999, 148–49).

When we choose to connect with the universal energy of Love, it is one way to sustain a caring-healing consciousness and a graceful intentionality to be in right relation with self/other and our situations in the midst of complex systems, be they human others or institutions. Transpersonal Caring Consciousness unites us with the energy of higher consciousness and opens space for a transcendent experience that transcends the negative lower vibration of energy. Daily simple contemplative practices, such as silence, breath work meditation, gratitude, and reading inspired texts and literature, help us sustain the shift to a higher frequency of light consciousness.

To capture the daily life of nurses and nursing caring phenomena, the ten Caritas Processes® within the Theory of Transpersonal Caring (Watson 2008, 2012) provide the language of the phenomenon of Unitary Human Caring; they become an entrée into sustaining higher consciousness and practicing human caring and healing.

Within the transpersonal theory, Caritas consciousness transcends time, space, and physicality—thus, consciousness is nonlocal. That is, Caritas-way-of-being is not localized in the mind or the ego. It resides in the unitary field—thus it is within Era III–Paradigm III: unitary awareness. Caritas Consciousness is opening energetically to the infinite field of universal Love as human consciousness evolves. Thus, a transpersonal caring moment is a mutually shared consciousness field experience, which can potentiate a healing moment in that it becomes part of the life history of each person and of the larger complex pattern of life and the universe (Watson 2012).

The Ten Caritas Processes® (2017) Affirmed as Universals of Human Caring

The named and researched human caring phenomena, ten Caritas Processes, have served as a philosophical-ethical theoretical guide to nursing caring-healing practices, both nationally and globally. These processes are considered universals of human caring, informed by the values and unitary worldview of caring science. A general summary of each process follows.

1. Sustaining humanistic-altruistic values by practicing loving-kindness, compassion, and equanimity with self/other
2. Being authentically present—enabling faith, hope, belief
3. Being sensitive to self and others by cultivating one's own spiritual practices—beyond ego to transpersonal presence
4. Developing and sustaining loving, trusting, caring relationships

5. Allowing for expression of positive and negative feelings—listening authentically to another person's story

6. Creatively problem-solving—"solution-seeking" through caring processes

7. Engaging in transpersonal teaching and learning within the context of a caring relationship; staying within the other's frame of reference

8. Creating a healing environment at all levels, a subtle environment for energetic, authentic caring practice

9. Reverentially assisting with basic needs as sacred acts; sustaining human dignity

10. Opening to the spiritual, mystery, unknowns—allowing for miracles.

Finally, caring science and the ten Caritas Processes and their prominent presence and evolution in educational and practice models worldwide invite a new discourse about the relationship between Caritas-Veritas Literacy Processes and unitary caring science as a manifestation of the unfolding maturing of nursing *eupraxis* within the Unitary Transformative paradigm. This evolved unitary science is both scientific and humanitarian; it intersects with the arts and humanities and related fields of study and practices, such as eco-caring, peace studies, philosophy, ethics, women/feminist studies, theology, education, and mind-body-spirit medicine and the growing field of integrative medicine and integrative nursing.

In conclusion, this chapter offered an overview of the evolution of caring science/Caritas Processes and the Theory of Transpersonal Human Caring over the past thirty-plus years. A historic view of the location of "caring" within the intellectual discourse of the nursing paradigm was explored, along with current thinking, which reconciled Caring Science Theory and the Unitary Science of Humans, resulting in Caritas-Veritas Literacy toward unitary caring science praxis/*eupraxis*—that is, "good in and of itself as a moral good" for self and society.

Summary: Discipline-Specific Caring Science Caritas Principles

At this point, the disciplinary discourse, consistent with caring science (Caritas and transpersonal), has matured to conclude that:

- Nursing phenomena are a unified whole.
- Nursing is caring within the human health (*healing*) experience.
- Nursing's most mature disciplinary concepts are located within a Unitary Transformative paradigm.
- Professional nursing's ethical-moral covenant with humanity includes Caritas-Veritas Literacy, honoring all of the vicissitudes of wholeness, consciousness, and human health (healing) experiences.

Then

- Nursing is an evolved, moral-ethical, unitary basic science discipline, distinct from conventional biomedical science, thus: unitary caring science.

CHAPTER FOUR

The Unitary Quantum Shift

New Consciousness as Guide to Disciplinary Development

The breeze at dawn has secrets to tell you.
  Don't go back to sleep.
You must ask for what you really want,
  Don't go back to sleep.
People are going back and forth across the doorsill
  Where the two worlds touch.
The door is round and open.
  Don't go back to sleep.
  RUMI (IN BARKS 1997, 36)

There is so much we do not know. Yet we stay consumed with the outer world of data science and separation of our "being/belonging" as our human-universe reality. Society promotes fear, designed to make us spend our precious life energy in ego wars, keeping us distracted and detoured from the beauty and quiet of our inner world—another reality that returns us to the infinity of universal love, that which unites us with all living things. It is that place we all know deep inside and that we long to return to. This is a time for nursing to wake up and "not go back to sleep."

This is a time for opening, surrendering, embracing, dancing joyfully, humbly, playfully, experientially, intellectually, academically, practically, into the sacred circle of it all. This is a time to not go quietly into the dark.

This is a time for all levels of nursing to awaken to the gifts we have to offer to humanity, a humanity that is crying out for life-giving, life-receiving practices/praxis, politics, and policies—authentic, morally informed human-universe caring and healing—for self, systems, institutions, and our world.

This shift moves my work from Caritas (caring and Love) to Veritas (truth seeking) through unitary caring science and a search for the good—*eupraxis*.

The irony and the gift is that once you wake up, you can't go back to sleep; you are called forward with the tide of life itself and deeper learning. You/we know another way, and y/our heart(s) will not let you/us regress.

So, once you step into unitary caring science, it is addictive and nourishing to your heart and soul. Once you enter and stay on the path of light, what unfolds is a continued enlightenment, a luminosity into another level of existence; we awaken to the beauty within and begin to "see" anew, pursuing meaningful, purposeful relations and work, asking new questions about why we are here. What are my gifts and talents? What am I to offer in service to the world?

> It does not matter how long you have waited, when you are ready, it is the time.
>
> BUDDHA

If and when you/we are ready, then we are free to embrace a new view of science, of our world, our universe. We realize that we can re-enchant, re-spirit our world; we can *sacramentalize* each moment, even in the midst of profane, materialistic corporate cultures. We practice gratitude for each gift of life—we embrace beauty, truth, honesty, creativity, poetry, music, literature, drama, and art; we see the holy in the midst of the profane. These gifts, too, are all part of unitary caring science; they come when we wake up and enter that which comes from the human spirit, the heart and soul of our one precious life. This consciousness shift invites us into miracles, mystery, unknowns, paradox, ambiguity, mysticism, prayer, faith, trust, gratitude, blessings, and soul care.

We are living, working, and even dying in institutions that are modeled on an industrial era of machines, products, and parts when we are faced with living in a quantum universe. When we understand the inhumane words, work, politics, and practices perpetuated by the outer competitive, corporate ego world, we have no choice but to wake up and *not go back to sleep* lest we all self-destruct out of ignorance—ignoring the very nature of life itself.

So here, in maturing the disciplinary foundation of nursing, we get to intellectually, academically, emotionally, experientially, and spiritually enter into and learn more about unitary caring science as another way forward. The irony is that nurses and nursing have had this unitary caring knowing all along, silently, behind the scenes. However, throughout history it has taken about 100 years for a profession to mature into a distinct discipline, with clarity of its phenomena and raison d'être.

We have reached a closer point in our maturing, knowing there is no end to it—our phenomena of human-universe are unfolding and evolving with us, infinite energy fractal fields within fields.

We are entering a quantum universe. These changes include physics and basic sciences and other scientific fields, and in spite of nursing's covenant with humanity and all it means to be human, we still often find ourselves locked in outdated thinking within a separatist-material-physical world ontology and an outer worldview as our starting point.

Unitary caring science, in contrast, has as its starting point a relational unitary ontology that honors the fact that we are all connected and that we *belong to the source*—the universal consciousness, spirit, infinite field of Universal Love—before and after the human plane of worldly experiences. Unitary caring science makes more explicit that unity and connectedness exist among all things in the great circle of life: change, illness, suffering, death, and rebirth. A unitary caring science orientation moves humanity closer to a moral community, closer to peaceful relationships with self and other communities—nations, states, other worlds, and time. Unitary caring science also unites us with the non-physical, the spirit work, the soul of self and science alike.

Unitary Caring Science—Ethic of Belonging

The starting point for Unitary Caring Science is based on the Ethic of Belonging, beginning with the belief and perennial wisdom of universal humanity—that our human experiences and journey through life and death are shared with all humanity across the globe. Human beings and the planet are united across time and space, belonging to the great sea of humanity.

An Ethic of Belonging was developed by the French philosopher Emmanuel Levinas (1969), who posited that our ethical worldview and starting point is the first principle of science. An Ethic of Belonging comes before the ontology of separate being; it acknowledges ethically, morally, and practically that we all belong to the infinite field of Universal Cosmic Love. We all come from this source of infinite Cosmic Love, and we all return to the infinite source, Cosmic Love—the mystery of life. This locates our worldview of unity within the sacred circle of life-death.

In academic terms, unitary caring science is an extant, evolved unitary model of science, grounded in a moral-ethical unitary ontological praxis that promotes, preserves, and sustains human dignity, wholeness, caring-healing, and health for all.

While Unitary Caring Science is trans-disciplinary, it is derived from the evolved discipline of nursing. Unitary Caring Science serves as a starting point for nursing and also for other health sciences as well as other fields, such as education and human service work. It reintroduces spirit and sacred dimensions back into our work, life, and world. It allows for a reunion between metaphysics and the material-physical world of modern science. Science and spirit unite in Unitary Caring Science. This worldview applies to all of humanity as we awaken to the emerging worldview necessary for the survival of humanity and Mother Earth.

Without having the paradigm-disciplinary clarity of what counts as science, guided by informed moral-philosophical values, nursing education, research, and scholarship will be sorely lacking in any new knowledge or understanding of the phenomena of human caring-healing, health, and evolving human consciousness. Nursing can certainly operate within Paradigms I and II, but if our consciousness remains there, nursing remains stuck in a worldview that is drastically changing in science and human consciousness. If nursing and nurses fail to evolve into Unitary Caring Consciousness, nursing may survive, but nurses will simply be very good technicians in a totally transformed quantum world.

Humanity is entering a new consciousness of unity, a reality that we are all connected on Mother Earth. Without preparation in the unitary caring science paradigm to address our phenomena and reason for existing, no progress is made in nursing fulfilling its social, moral, scientific responsibility to humanity. Nursing's focus on wholeness, caring, consciousness, and unitary views of human-universe prepares nurses and nursing to provide voice, knowledge, and informed moral action—praxis—in service to humankind.

Background for this emerging worldview includes a greater awareness of the metaphysical, the unexplainable phenomena—the ineffable. When we enter Unitary Caring Science, we are reminded that data are not information, information is not knowledge, knowledge is not understanding, understanding is not wisdom (Watson 2005). Information alone does not lead to knowing or wise knowing. The phenomenon of wise knowing is what Patti Lather called "groking" (Lather 2010, 89), from Robert Heinlein's *Stranger in a Strange Land*

(1961). *Groking* is from the Martian language, meaning an internalized way of knowing. Nursing unitary scholar Marlaine Smith (1992b) posited that all knowledge is actually personal knowledge/knowing, again affirming Parker Palmer's thesis of "epistemology as ethic." Likewise, Patricia Munhall (1993) called for a way of knowing that is "unknowing"—unlearning or "non-knowing"—as an important place to be for reflection and knowledge-wisdom development. This view highlights our need to unlearn the outdated paradigms of previous eras of thinking and human evolution.

In the Buddhist philosophy, there is the notion of *"the don't know mind"*—a very good place to be. If we think we know, then there is no space to learn anything new. This view of knowing and non-knowing, emptying out, is akin to Caritas-Veritas, which allows for unknowns, mysteries, and miracles. In the metaphysical work of healing we can call this experience non-local, mystical, or spiritual, beyond the physical-empirical ways of knowing and being in the world. Ken Wilber (2000), a visionary philosopher whose works have impacted our world of science and knowledge for more than three decades, reminds us that the teachings of the world's greatest yogis, saints, and sages were and are trans-rational—that is, all contemplative traditions aim at going within and beyond reason. They adhere to the notion that truth is the result of personal experience (Wilber 2000, 271), that these truths and this "no-knowing" form of knowing are open to everyone who wishes to explore/experiment/experience and thus disclose for themselves the truth or falsity of non-rational claims. These claims are consistent with caring-healing phenomena and human caring experiences. This form of unknowing/non-knowing exists in higher domains of awareness of evolution and directly embraces experiences such as love, compassion, beauty, identity, reality, self, truth, and meaning. This higher-domain way of knowing is based on hundreds of years of experimental introspection and communal verification (Wilber 2000, 273).

These historical communal verification criteria, valid across the centuries, are translated into "inter-subjective confirmability" in contemporary research language. Inter-subjectivity is a valid criterion to incorporate in qualitative research. When others validate from within and agree, there is a sense of "knowing." For example, the "truth" of the story or narrative of the phenomenon is validated through general consensus by others. Inner communal truth rings "true" or captures a truth or essence of the phenomenon in question. This is Veritas, so-called truth, as validation from within.

Lather's view of groking can also be known as wisdom, a knowing that embraces the whole person's learning and knowing. Also, this groking captures "a knowing" that is already known and is a given "on the face of it"; however, this is often not acknowledged or explored in a conventional mind-set. These areas move into metaphysical phenomena, even though the notion of metaphysical is not addressed in mainstream thinking in research, philosophy, or science.

Since unitary caring science inverts the paradigm, it breaks into new territory within a mature evolutionary view of philosophy, science, and humanity—an upward model of science, open to embrace mystery and miracles and even the mystical: spiritual experiences as a form of truth. When we invert the paradigm we challenge, if not en/lighten, the dominant perspective.

As noted earlier, while caring is a means to a curing end, when we invert it we acknowledge that *caring is also an end in and of itself.* As such, human caring (and Caritas/love) becomes the highest moral-ethical commitment we can make to humanity and ourselves (influenced by Sally Gadow). This perspective is now captured as an evolved Caritas-Veritas within the transpersonal theory and philosophy of human caring and new views of Unitary Caring Science Praxis.

This worldview invites and is open to deeply introspective human experiences and even metaphysical-spiritual phenomena, which people around the globe have known for thousands of years. Disciplinary-focused education and research on unitary caring science adheres to the paradigm in which it is located: unitary worldview/cosmology. This evolution is grounded in a meaningful philosophical-ethical, epistemological-methodological context for practice/praxis and healthcare policy—policy guided by a unitary worldview and principles underpinned by core Caritas-Veritas values.

The discipline of nursing is what holds nursing's timeless values, its heritage and traditions, and its knowledge development toward sustaining humanity and health for all.

- The discipline is what holds and honors an ontology of the whole person—the unity of mind-body-spirit and a relational unitary worldview.
- The discipline is what adheres to nursing's philosophical orientation toward humanity and nursing's ethical global covenant with humanity to sustain human caring-healing-health for all.
- The discipline is what holds the theories, the orientation toward knowledge development, and what counts as knowledge—expanding conventional medical epistemologies.
- The discipline is what holds nursing's research traditions and diverse and evolving approaches to knowledge development; the discipline-specific orientation to knowledge critiques what counts as knowledge.
- The discipline addresses expanded, diverse, creative, and innovative methodologies and methods consistent with human caring-healing-health/illness experiences and phenomena.
- The discipline holds grand, middle-range, and situation-specific theories to provide a shared evolved, unitary worldview whereby health is related to social-moral justice and whole person/whole system processes and outcomes, acknowledging that human caring and eco-caring are one—for example, humans and planet are connected. This reflects a distinct disciplinary position.

It is generally expected that the disciplinary knowledge of any field is what informs and matures the professional practice. The disciplinary matrix of Unitary Caring is what holds the meta-paradigm, the values, the metaphysics, the philosophical-moral meta-framework with respect to what it means to be human; the discipline's values of truth and honor embrace the unity of being-belonging—acknowledging the oneness of mind-body-spirit/universe. The discipline is what frames the focus of, and a distinct perspective on, the subject matter; the discipline holds the theories and research traditions.

Any profession whose disciplinary context lacks clarity loses its way in the midst of the outer-worldly changes and forces designed to conform to the institutional status quo of the moment. All too often our educational practices and research perpetuate an outmoded, unenlightened profession without groking the discipline. Once nurse educators, researchers, practitioners, and administrators *know* the disciplinary worldview, true transformation occurs from within. Unitary caring science then becomes the foundational ethical-ontological starting point for nursing education, patient care, research, leadership, and administrative practices.

UNITARY CARING SCIENCE CONTEXT FOR NURSING EDUCATION

- Knowledge of caring cannot be assumed; it is an epistemic-ethical-theoretical endeavor that requires ongoing explication and development.

- Unitary Caring Science is grounded in a relational, ethical ontology of unity within the universe that informs the epistemology, methodology, pedagogy, and praxis of caring in nursing and related fields.

- Unitary Caring Science embraces epistemological pluralism; it questions the status quo of what counts as knowledge and how knowledge is known; it uncovers and reveals Palmer's thesis of "epistemology as ethic," seeking to understand the dominant dated worldview of knowledge and opening up the intersection and underdeveloped connections between the arts and humanities and the clinical caring sciences.

- Unitary Caring Science embraces all ways of knowing/being/doing/becoming/belonging—ethical, intuitive, personal, empirical, and aesthetic—allowing spiritual/metaphysical, mystical, unknown ways of knowing and being, transcending being.

• Unitary Caring Science inquiry encompasses methodological pluralism, whereby the method flows from the phenomenon of concern—diverse forms of inquiry seek to unify ontological, philosophical, ethical, and theoretical views while incorporating empirics and technology.

Unitary Caring Nursing Education

Nursing education and curriculum guided by Unitary Caring Science introduces and implements emancipatory pedagogies using the full range of the arts, humanities, literature, personal stories, and inner subjective meanings that integrate clinical technical knowledge within the context of the unitary field. The teaching-learning methodologies help students learn about nursing intellectually and experientially from a unitary caring science worldview. For example, clinical learning and classrooms-laboratories create a culture and community of human caring and healing—Communitas in action—a human studio model of learning about energy, the artistry of being human, self-caring, meditative-contemplative practices, and transpersonal relations in and out of the classroom.

Unitary Caring Science pedagogies would include an environment for authentic dialogue, as well as continual opportunities for caring practice (*eupraxis*). Pedagogical practice would include a safe space for honest, constructive, appreciative forms of inquiry and feedback—critiquing (*dyspraxia*) practices in a safe space and a trusting relational environmental field. Pedagogical Communitas circles would be used for active, engaged learning for moral Caritas-Veritas Literacy and ontological development, transcending technological development alone.

Practitioners would study unitary principles, theories, the phenomenon of wholeness, patients' families' subjective experiences, and patterns of health. Students and faculty alike would explore self-learning, self-caring, and contemplative approaches to growth and insight beyond facts and knowledge per se. There would be an environment of intellectual curiosity and a search for moral as well as scientific truths.

The curriculum would be framed around knowledge of nursing theories, exploring all ways of knowing about a given clinical-human phenomenon—for example, the phenomena of suffering, healing, transpersonal human caring relations, patterns, community, consciousness, unitary wholeness, and the relational ethics of belonging—as a guide to knowledgeable, informed moral practices. Nursing practices would be geared toward energetic, holistic caring-healing modalities, a full integration of the technological and ontological literacy of Caritas and Veritas moral values.

For example, the nursing education curriculum would follow these disciplinary elements:

- **Ethic of Belonging** as entrance into Unitary Caring Science; this opens up a curriculum and learning culture that invites a critique of the dominant medical-clinical-institutional paradigm, which separates human-environment oneness, reveals social-moral injustices, and perpetuates culturally unsafe practices.
- **Ontology of oneness-wholeness**—Students learn that the human-environment universe is the focus of global human caring-healing issues. This worldview is lived out in the classrooms, and a culture of social-moral justice, safety, and Caritas-Veritas Literacy is manifest.
- **Expanding epistemologies**—Invites all ways of knowing in exploring, inquiring, and appreciating research on any phenomenon; leads students to use the full range of knowing, including wise knowing; faculty have Caritas-Veritas Literacy as their guide for teaching-learning, thus honoring the whole student learning from within, knowing and appreciating that students have different learning styles.

- **The ten Caritas-Veritas Processes** serve as one exemplar of how to structure caring science learning experiences, curricula, and guides to authentic personal/professional learning. Core concepts of health, wellness, being-becoming, caring, and healing are explored using patients' experiences, theories, and various worldviews.

- **Methodological wholeness**—Learning experiences invite multiple and creative forms of inquiry; they encourage students to draw upon their own backgrounds to use existing and creative new forms of inquiry that are ontologically consistent with the phenomena of inquiry and interest. These diverse methods can generate new forms of knowing and new knowledge of caring-healing-health phenomena. Drama, art, music, poetry, theater, film, personal stories, photography, documentaries, clinical phenomena, and literature are woven into methods of inquiry as liberating learning methods, beyond didactic, cognitive, content-laden, "banking information" learning methods.

- In the **digital world of online learning,** rather than view space as distancing, see it as connecting, creating a Caritas-Communitas platform to inspire others for a shared unitary consciousness. This approach affirms that the faculty's entire caring consciousness transcends time, space, and physicality (Watson 2008); therefore, students experience a community of caring as a unifying culture of the classroom or the computer.

- **Pedagogy-androgyny**—Emancipatory, liberating approaches to teaching-learning would be geared toward a faculty-student Caritas-Communitas culture; would draw upon multiple ways of learning and teaching methods; and would focus on self-learning, self-caring, self-knowledge, self-control, well-being/becoming, and approaches to self-healing.

- **Theories of nursing** within the discipline will be the guides for learning. Any assignment of a phenomenon of study would draw upon all ways of knowing: for example, personal, intuitive, empirical, aesthetic, ethical, experimental, and technical, including metaphysical-spiritual learning, also leading to new forms of praxis and policy. The classroom and clinical experiences would attend to aesthetics and appeal to the higher senses.

- The **content of the curriculum** is structured around teaching styles that meet the complex needs of individuals and their learning styles, backgrounds, and cultural views. The teaching method would also include contemplative centering, reflective and reflexive practices, and exercises/assignments for self-learning and spiritual growth.

- **Praxis**—This is where Caritas-Veritas is lived out through informed moral literacy actions in which knowing/doing/being/becoming are lived out in the moment as one art/act. This is where basic disciplinary Unitary Caring Science principles of presence, intentionality, caring consciousness, energetic field, and the transpersonal caring moment can authentically be manifest as various levels of eupraxis—unitary caring science praxis. It is here that we teach and implement Caritas-Veritas as ontological competencies/literacies. This is where ontological design projects can be co-created between academic and clinical settings. This is where transformations of self and system work together to transform from the inside out. New models are created and implemented as, it is hoped, models for humanity and our world.

See appendix B for current ontological projects of caring science.

CHAPTER FIVE

From Ontological Competencies to Caritas-Veritas Literacy*

Caritas Quote

While the meaning of literacy is associated with the abilities to read and write, the notion of having fluency in caring at both personal and professional levels introduces new meaning to deepen our ways of attending to and cultivating how to *Be* deeply human/humane, and how to *Be-caring* and have a healing presence.

Such literacy includes an evolved and continually evolving emotional heart intelligence, consciousness and intentionality and level of sensitivity and efficacy, followed by a continuing lifelong process and journey of self-growth and self-awareness.

This level of evolved Being/Ontological presence is now ethically required for any professional engaged in caring-healing. (Watson 2008b, 23–24)

---

* Some sections of this chapter are extracted and modified from Watson 2017; used with permission.

This chapter highlights my expanding views of Caritas and Caritas Literacy as a way of being/knowing/becoming/evolving as humans and as a "universal humanity"—one world/one heart—whereby we awaken to the ethical and scientific fact that our *being Caritas for self and other* is affecting the universal consciousness of all of life and the planet earth. It outlines some of the basic dynamics and meaning of Caritas and Caritas Literacy, as well as an evolved "Critical Caritas Literacy" as the moral, ethical, and scientific counterpoint to a kind of "illiteracy." Literacy and praxis go together in terms of Caritas-Veritas, in that a moral commitment is underlying the timeless, enduring purity of values of goodness, truth, and love that nursing praxis and unitary caring bring to our world. The counterpoint to Caritas-Veritas in action, we witness an institutional, professional preoccupation with technological, cognitive, task-conscious competencies, void of our shared human life world—we diminish or totalize a shared unified world of learning, growing, evolving as caring-loving humans in service to our world, sustaining humanity and our survival on planet earth. Once Caritas-Veritas Literacy is uncovered, it becomes the basis for understanding Caritas-Veritas as an enduring professional guide for living out and sustaining Unitary Caring Science Praxis.

Literacy is seemingly a term everyone knows. However, even though it has many meanings, literacy usually refers to the basic cognitive skills of reading and writing and numeracy-numbers—counting and manipulation. Nevertheless, in the "history of literacy in English, the word 'literate' meant to be 'familiar with literature' or more generally 'well educated, learned.' Ironically, over time it was reduced to [the] ability to read and write" (unesco.org 2008, 147).

Scholars have debated and critiqued various definitions of literacy and have challenged and expanded the limited meanings of the term. These expansive views are constantly emerging, leading to expanding visions and new questions and understandings of "being" literate and "becoming" perhaps more "literate" at an expanded human consciousness level. A literate person is one who is able to access and process information, knowledge, images, and symbols and to reflect, critique, and interpret meaning—even construct meaning. Being literate extends to the ability to incorporate concrete experience, experiential learning, contexts, and situations into one's life field—a form of wisdom. Thus, the term *literacy* has evolved to incorporate the fact that there are multiple literacies.

Indeed, as the notions of literacy have expanded, perhaps we also have ways of being in which some collective institutional mind-sets could be considered "illiterate."

Journey to Caring Science and Caritas-Veritas Literacy

Synchrony Sidebar

While writing this book between January and August 2017, in mid-August I discovered that Dr. Joyce Perkins, a Watson Caring Science postdoctoral scholar, was writing along parallel and intersecting lines. This synchrony and so-called coincidence is a living example of the unitary field and how two writers without overt, verbal, or written communication are arriving at similar positions regarding unitary caring science and the expansion of Caritas Processes. While they are similar in direction, the two differ in context of meaning and focus. Perkins uses the term *virtue* as a value component to help to redefine Caritas within Unitary Caritas emergence (Perkins 2017).

I use the term *Veritas* to capture the Aristotle meaning of praxis with a moral values commitment component, which becomes a form of Caritas-Veritas Literacy. We both explored the evolution of the terms carative (Paradigm I, Watson 1970) to transpersonal caring (Paradigm II and quasi-III, Watson 1985) to Caritas Processes (Paradigm II, quasi-III, Watson 2008, 2012).

Carative-Caritas Evolution from Paradigm I to Paradigm III

In my first book (Watson 1979) I used the term *Carative Factors* to capture the meaning of caring in contrast to curative. Carative Factors can now easily be seen as Paradigm I. After my personal growth and inner journey, I transposed Carative Factors to Caritas

Process, the evolution of Paradigm II. With this shift I was intentionally moving beyond the denser energy language of carative. Paradigm II Caritas had higher-vibration energy, bringing love and healing and a higher level of consciousness as the core of human caring. Now I make another turn toward unitary caring science—Paradigm III more explicitly.

Caritas is a journey to the heart of our professional practice and the heart of our humanity. So what do we mean by Caritas Literacy?

As emphasized in earlier chapters, the original Aristotle Greek meaning of praxis has two explicit components: *moral action* associated with values and *commitment to moral actions*. This book incorporates all my previous scholarship; however, it has a more evolved unitary consciousness. *Here, praxis is defined as informed moral unitary caring practice*—practice informed by a shared, evolved, discipline-specific, unitary consciousness combined with the onto-logical-ethical-epistemological moral comportment that has historically underpinned nursing actions across time.

Here, in unitary caring science philosophy and praxis, I evoke Veritas along with Caritas to convey the morally committed Aristotelian meaning of praxis. Veritas represents and names the purity of nursing virtues and values of enduring truth, beauty, honor, and dignity—all associated with unitary caring science. Caritas remains core to my previous theoretical-philosophical writings (Watson 2008, 2012) to capture universals of deep authentic caring, including love. However, now Veritas is used with Caritas to convey the timeless universal moral foundation of caring and love for praxis. Sometimes we need language to provide additional meaning to what we already know but that passes us by.

The term *Caritas* is from Latin, referring to that which is precious and cannot be taken for granted; it conveys charity in the sense of use of self in compassionate service to humankind. From my writings (Watson 2008, 2012), I use Caritas to depict the deeper ethical philosophical value foundation of authentic professional human caring practice. Caring Science encompasses all the complexities and vicissitudes of humanity; the term *Caritas* encompasses loving consciousness as the core of human caring—deepening the meaning of professional nurse caring beyond the outer slogan and trite use of the term *caring*, which has become commonplace and even commercialized as a commodity to be bought and sold. Thus Caritas and Unitary Caring Science are grounded in and founded on a deep ethical-moral philosophical way of being/becoming more human/humane: a human evolving in higher/deeper consciousness toward connection with the source—Universal Love.

This mode of literacy of Caritas-Veritas invites a total transformation of self and systems. In this model of Unitary Caring Science, the changes occur not from the outer focus on systems. Changes come from that deep inner place, emerging within and aligning with the creativity and divine flow of the human spirit. Here is where the deep humanity, the individual heart and consciousness of practitioners, evolves and connects with the ultimate source of all true re-formation/transformation. This becomes a living Caritas-Veritas Literacy for advancing Unitary Caring Science Praxis.

By integrating Caritas with Veritas, we come closer to affirming the values of virtue and goodness, moral truths, ideals of preserving and sustaining humanity and human dignity/integrity, allowing for the evolution of humans to touch infinity—to bring more light/love into our daily life world. This literacy reaches to the highest level of consciousness—reaching for the beloved, the divine, the infinite unitary field of Cosmic Love. This infinite consciousness evolution—posed by Levinas (1969), Teilhard de Chardin (1959, 1964), Hawkins (2002), and others—is the very opposite of totalizing humanity. Without Caritas-Veritas Literacy consciousness, we are in danger of reducing others to the moral status of object and cutting off their own source for self-renewal, for the soul connection allowing for infinite evolution closer to the divine–infinite love (Levinas 1969).

Without evolving toward a unitary ontological, Veritas moral literacy, we can be cruel and insensitive to self and others. We become instruments for institutional biocidic practices and inhumane, disparate levels of care for different people, races, and standings. We contribute to moral and social injustices, something that dis-spirits us from our own humanity.

Critical Literacy for Unitary Caring Science

The vision of multiple literacies has opened the horizon to identify language literacy as an instrument of power and oppression, for example, considering dominant discourses and use of language, which endangers cultures and local knowledge. This postmodern critique of literacy was heavily influenced by Paolo Freire (1972, 2014 [1995]) and the notion of "critical literacy." His writings and work moved the conversation about and use of the terms *literate* and *literacy* beyond the task-conscious, conventional basic meaning of reading and writing.

For example, Freire integrated notions of active learning within socio-cultural settings. His pedagogical goal was to engage with books and written texts but also to engage through "reading"—that is, interpreting, reflecting on, interrogating, theorizing, investigating, exploring, probing, and questioning and writing: acting on and dialogically transforming the world. He also highlighted the fact that the words people use to give meaning to their lives are created and conditioned by the world they inhabit.

So by introducing and integrating the terms *Caritas Literacy* and *Caritas-Veritas Literacy* into praxis, we make a conceptual, moral, and philosophical leap to a new level of moral actions geared to transform the world. This evolved notion of a critical literacy view is tied to praxis (*eupraxis*) in that it conveys the original Aristotelian moral value component, making explicit that Caritas-Veritas Literacy is one underlying principle of praxis and demonstrating through moral informed actions a commitment to liberating and bettering humankind in the world.

This form of Caritas-Veritas Literacy can be translated into the life world of nursing and nurses. Nurses live in a subjective inner world motivated by heart-centered human-to-human caring as a moral ideal and an ethical philosophical imperative, yet nurses inhabit an institutional world conditioned by a medical-scientific-clinical view of caring literacy as consisting of concrete medical tasks and cognitive rational skills, separate from their inner life world and authentic self. So the meaning of "literacy" as used in the institutional clinical world of nursing (which can be considered illiterate in some respects) is inconsistent with the evolution of "critical literacy" within Freire's worldview.

Likewise, literacy in the mainstream industrial world differs from Caritas-Vertias Literacy, which is concerned with critical reflections on praxis and what praxis brings to our discourse. Do we offer *eupraxis* to our world, or do we contribute to *dyspraxia*?

- Does our current healthcare (sick-care) system address or even ask the question about what it means to be an evolved, literate human being?
- What does it mean to sustain humanity?
- What does it mean to practice human caring authentically and morally?
- What does it mean to care?
- What does it mean to heal?
- What does it mean to be healthy? To be well? To become well?

These are all rhetorical, ethical value questions that inform our discourse on the concept of literacy. The questions inform so-called *moral values literacy*. More specifically, these provocative, probing, evocative, evolving moral questions underlie the Caritas-Veritas Literacy that informs or deforms nursing practice/praxis. Thus, we can begin to see the difference between conventional practice literacy (reduced to tasks and skills of doing or cognately knowing) and praxis literacy—literacy that is informed by both knowledge and moral, timeless, enduring values. Thus Caritas-Veritas Literacy is uncovered as the critical discourse in guiding us to unitary caring science praxis.

The evolution of the concept of "critical literacy" and the critique of skill-task literacy is reinforced by the writings of the French philosopher Michel Foucault (1980, 1984), a popular postmodern social theorist and literary critic. Foucault's social-political critique of dominant institutional standards and discourses revealed and reflected how language and discourse control and oppress versus liberate.

Foucault introduced the entire notion of "text" and "discourse" to critique literacy within wider socio-political practices—for example, we can critique discourse in hospitals:

- What is the dominant discourse?
- What is the dominant language?
- What is the dominant text?
- What is the power structure?
- How is language constructed to control and dominate health and human behavior?
- What and who holds the dominant power?
- Whose language controls the discourse?

Critical Caritas-Veritas Literacy

Critical literacy is close to Caritas-Veritas Literacy as it has evolved within Caring Science and Unitary Caring Science Praxis. This evolution of the term *literate* invites understandings of being and becoming "literate" in ways that relate to critical reflection and the capacity to deepen and critique cultural, ethical, humane social justice views and policies, affecting an understanding of what it means to be human. The Caritas-Veritas Literate human is morally informed and has capacity beyond task-conscious learning and basic-survival living toward an evolved, heart-centered, loving unitary ontological consciousness for purposive learning and living.

Critical Caritas-Veritas Literacy asks new questions at the "I level":

- What does it mean to me to be/become an evolved human?
- How do I practice and sustain caring and compassion toward self and others?

- How can I continue to question and evolve to a higher level of loving, caring, forgiving consciousness, contributing to caring and healing for self and others and Mother Earth?
- What morally informed Caritas-Veritas–conscious acts could I engage in today (privately, secretly, or in public) to be in right authentic relation with others and myself and my environment?
- What would change if I began my day considering that this is the last day of my life? Or a new beginning—to dwell in humility, surrender to a higher purpose, an inner guide? Trusting in the universe and that which is greater than me?
- What would happen if I dwell in silence for even five minutes?
  - Be quiet for five minutes and see what happens.
- Can I simply breathe into this moment, knowing that this is all there is: this moment?
  - All I have are moments—can I be present to this transpersonal now, a transpersonal caring moment, as an *eternal now* . . . just as it is?

Critical Caritas-Veritas Literacy ultimately comes from within each person's subjective inner life world, morally aroused for reflective and contemplative self-growth, self-caring experiences that contribute to the whole of humanity. Within this framework of Caritas-Veritas Literacy, it is important to realize that the nurse is not only *in* the environment, able to make significant changes in ways of being/doing/knowing in the physical environment, but that the *nurse IS the environment* (Quinn 1992; Watson 2005).

Thus, the nurse is invited to engage in significant insight into the *nurse-self* as a moral value—a good in and of itself, a conscious energetic-vibrational field of consciousness and intentionality that affects the entire environment, for better or for worse. The nurse's (caring-loving) consciousness radiates a higher vibrational frequency of light (Zukav 1990). A nurse without an informed, "literate" caring value consciousness can actually be "biocidic"—that is, toxic, life-destroying, and destructive to the experience of others (Halldorsdottir 1991). In contrast, a nurse who is cultivating onto-logical competencies in Caritas-Veritas Literacy is more likely to be "biogenic"—that is, life-giving and life-receiving for self and others and thereby more likely to engage in and experience transpersonal caring-healing moments. As the nurse cultivates these ontological literate abilities and sensitivities of Caritas-Veritas Literacy, there is an invitation to open to inner healing processes and praxis that expand to infinite new possibilities.

The ontological Caritas-Veritas Literate nurse mediates between technological competencies and the emotional-intellectual human needs of others. The Caritas-Veritas Literate nurse is the intersec-tion between the depersonalized, totalizing other versus the preser-vation of humanity and dignity, honoring the wholeness of self and other. The morally informed literate nurse cultivates skills/praxis of being-caring/being Caritas/being-becoming Veritas—knowl-edge and morally informed values in action. Such exploration into the literacy of caring incorporates the ethical, philosophical, and theoretical foundations of professional caring-healing. This view of Caritas-Veritas Literacy serves as core whole person knowledge and deepens and affirms the original meaning of praxis. It leads directly back to the evolution of Transpersonal Caring Theory, the original Caring Science theory of Caritas Processes, to Caring Science as Sacred Science, to Caritas-Veritas Literacy as the basis for Unitary Caring Science Praxis.

> Knowledge of what is does not open the door directly to what should be.
>
> ALBERT EINSTEIN

> Why do we conform to what is, and is no longer working, without asking [moral] questions about what might be?
>
> SARTRE

Caritas-Veritas *Illiteracy*

To better our understanding of Critical Caritas-Veritas Literacy, it is perhaps helpful to analyze it against non–Caritas-Veritas Literacy: that is, *Caritas-Veritas Illiteracy.*

What Is versus What Could/Should Be

The counterpoint to Critical Caritas-Veritas Literacy within Unitary Caring Science is Caritas-Veritas Illiteracy—that is, inhumane task-conscious practices; use of lower-vibration, objectifying language; scientizing of human emotions and expressions; repressive, insensitive, dehumanizing, dividing-separating actions and policies; crafting a commodification of caring and people. Harsh, unkind, controlling cultures within impersonal institutions, corporations, and social networks can be considered illiterate. For example, Caritas-Veritas illiteracy is devoid of purity of value for self/other; devoid of timeless, enduring virtues that guide reverence and the sacredness of life; devoid of the humility of mystery, awe, wonder at precious life; devoid of the "ethical demand" of realization that we hold another person's life in our hands (Logstrup 1997). The Caritas-Veritas illiterate person, or specifically an illiterate nurse, becomes a co-conspirator with a system that is discriminating, labeling, blaming, ostracizing, and totalizing the humanity of another—therefore totalizing one's own humanity and the unity of being/becoming.

Illiterate healthcare systems use distancing-depersonalizing language, which can be abusive; they use derogatory terms to reference "other," meaning someone who is different, of another color or race, from a foreign country, or poor and lacking resources. Such systems use this means of treatment or withholding treatment and care of "other" as a way to justify withholding that person's care and basic human needs and rights. In an illiterate healthcare system there is evidence of hard edge words and language, which separates, labels, diagnoses, divides, and conquers—inciting fear and distrust as a means of "control over" others. All these aspects of illiteracy in our healthcare and in society are a form of morally, ethically, and literally totalizing another's humanity. In the words of Levinas, we either support the infinite evolution of humanity-universe oneness or we cut off a human's possibility by reducing him or her to object status, to be controlled by outside illiterate social forces.

It takes an enduring, evolving literate human to critique and uncover the pathology of illiteracy in our world. That is why nursing's moral ideals of being of service to global humanity offer an ideal for moral leadership, making unitary connections between caring and peace. Caritas-Veritas Literacy, in all its shadow-light dimensions, all the vicissitudes of human existence, becomes the grounds for our being caring and respecting the wholeness of "other," even when that person differs from us.

Nursing is so greatly needed at this time because of Caritas-Veritas Literacy Consciousness, held in the moral purity blueprint of Veritas as a lasting moral guideline. The discipline of nursing with its Caritas-Veritas Literacy is needed to overcome moral institutional illiteracy in small and grand ways. Such illiteracy is not always known or seen; nevertheless, nurses are participating energetically in the moral Unitary Caring Science Praxis of re-patterning self and system, helping healthcare move from illiteracy to literacy in an effort to preserve global humanity, human caring, dignity, social justice, and health for all.

At this point in human history we are challenged to critique and re-pattern, if not transform, healthcare from illiteracy/ignorance about being human and humane—ignorance about the oneness of our universal humanity. Caritas-Veritas Literacy helps avoid reducing another to the moral status of an object. Caritas-Veritas Literacy resists participating in a system that allows another to be manipulated and controlled, depersonalized, totalized as "other." The Critical Caritas-Veritas Literate nurse and person honors and reveres our shared humanity—celebrating liberating, emancipatory learning, growing, and trusting through love; participating in and co-creating a living Caritas-Veritas Communitas for a global, morally literate humanity.

Critical Caritas-Veritas Literacy—Ontological Unitary Caring Science Praxis

This section offers a guide to overcome Caritas-Veritas Illiteracy—the dominant health institutional focus on medicalizing and objectifying humans, typified by a preoccupation with technological competencies and industrial measures and practices. Critical Caritas-Veritas Literacy not only critiques self, system, and society for Caritas Illiteracy but also poses another way to balance, repattern, transcend, and transform the dominant task-conscious illiterate human culture.

Educating the mind without educating the heart is no education at all.

ARISTOTLE

Critical Caritas-Veritas Literacy as Ontology

This translates into Caritas-Veritas—that is, a special way of being/living virtues and values as a loving, caring, compassionate human being—evolving to become more and more caring, kind, compassionate, and loving with self, others, and all living things. In my 2008 book I developed a section of ontological competencies and Caritas/Caring Literacy as the first level of development of this concept of Caritas Literacy. This concept was influenced by others, including Joan Boyce (2007) and faculty associates at the Watson Caring Science Institute. This has evolved to Caritas-Veritas Literacy as the basis for ontological competencies, moving from competencies to literacy.

Caritas-Veritas Literacy as a unitary ontology brings forth dimensions of the art and artistry of our being. It conveys an evolved and continually evolving health-heart intelligence, consciousness, and intentionality—a level of sensitivity and moral efficacy; a lifelong journey of self-healing, self-growth, and deliberate spiritual practices (Watson 2008, 22–23).

Such literacy includes an evolved and continually evolving emotional heart intelligence, consciousness, and intentionality and a level of sensitivity and efficacy, followed by a continuing awakening to the Infinity of Love. This awakening of one's being and abilities cultivates skills and awareness of holding, conveying, practicing, and communicating thoughts of caring, loving, kindness, equanimity, and so on, as part of one's professional being. This level of evolved being/ontological presence is now ethically required for any professional engaged in the caring-healing praxis.

Perhaps this requirement has always been present in the value/Veritas tradition of healing professions, but somewhere along the way professional education and practices took a detour from the value foundation of our shared humanity. A return to a focus on unitary ontological competencies/literacy seems essential to balance and carry out the pervasive technological competencies, helping to make these literacy skills, values, and ways of being-becoming more human as part of the requirements for nursing education and practice.

Watson's Caritas-Veritas Literacy Guide to Unitary Caring Science Praxis

- Cultivate personal caring consciousness and intentionality as a starting point.
- Suspend role and status; honor each person's unique and diverse gifts, talents, and contributions as essential to the whole.
- Speak and listen without judgment; know the difference between discerning and judging.
- Work from heart-centered consciousness with others, seeking shared meaning and common values.
- Listen with compassion and an open heart—without interrupting.
- Learn to be still, to center self while holding a "still point" inside in the midst of turmoil.

- Welcome and cultivate silence for reflection, contemplation, clarity.
- Caritas-Veritas Consciousness transcends ego; it is transpersonal, generating a new energetic field in the moment. This consciousness restores purity and the enduring, timeless virtue of love and kindness, and it creates a human-to-human, spirit-to-spirit connection with others. Life and work are divided no more; the personal becomes the professional (modified from Watson 2008, 25–26; Watson 2003, 201).

The following points serve as general unfinished ontological Caritas-Veritas Literacy guides:

- Pause before entering a patient's room.
- "Read" the energetic field when entering the life space/field of others.
- Cultivate the ability to *be authentically present*—be with—versus doing.
- Accurately identify self, and address the other person by name.
- Maintain eye contact as culturally and sensitively appropriate.
- Energetically ground self and other as comforting, soothing, calming acts.
- Accurately detect another's feelings.
- Stay within the other's frame of reference.
- Authentically *listen* to another person's story without interrupting or trying to "fix" anything, knowing that this moment of listening is a healing gift for both of you.
- Hold another in your heart space with unconditional compassion, kindness, dignity, and regard.
- Hold silence with another, creating open space for connecting, reflecting.
- Practice intentional use of loving touch—non-contact therapeutic touch (TT) and healing touch (HT), as well as intentional physical touch.

- Alter or re-pattern the environmental field with energetic consciousness shifts to a high-vibrational presence; attend to the physical environment for energy flow and removal of clutter, offering beauty and aesthetics in the space.

- Translate and carry out conventional nursing skills and tasks into conscious, intentional, literate (Caritas-Veritas) caring-healing acts—manifestations of unitary caring science praxis.

- Translate conventional actions into meaningful, intentional, literate caring-healing rituals.

- Incorporate healing arts and general and advanced caring-healing modalities and integrative practices into the culture of patient and system care.

- Discern, critique, and work constructively to re-pattern/transform the dominant culture of Caritas Illiteracy into a more enlightened, more open culture and system that radiates unitary caring science/Caritas-Veritas Literacy as the new norm for global caring-healing–health systems now and in the future.

Summary

The Latin word *Caritas* and ten Caritas Processes originally offered a new vocabulary to capture what are now considered universals of human caring. This language was also embedded in the unitary, moral, ontological-ethical perspective, allowing for new ways of thinking about caring and inviting a new image—even a metaphor—of caring-healing practices to develop.

In this unitary quantum era, nurses/practitioners can no longer let our morally committed virtues pass us by. We can morally and ethically no longer remain committed to conventional medicalized-clinical routines and industrial product-line views of nursing and healthcare (and humanity)—all contained within limited views of our life and death.

Simply put, Critical Caritas-Veritas Literacy begins with self being present and open to the purity of values to honor self and others; opening to compassion, mercy, gentleness, gratitude, loving-kindness, and equanimity toward and with self as beginning and end and the starting point of the same with others. Caritas-Veritas Literacy calls forth purity of values and the virtue of timeless, enduring moral values required to sustain global humanity and the ineffable gifts of beauty, wonder, awe, mystery, and miracles in our daily lives. Unitary caring science praxis, underpinned by Caritas-Veritas Literacy, "brings forth a love of humanity and all living things; the immanent, subtle, radiant, shadow and light vicissitudes of experiences along the way—honoring with reverence the mystery, paradox, ambiguity, the unknowns, the impermanence of all that inform and mold us with [the] pain and joy of it all" (Watson 2008, xviii).

The purpose of this book is to help self and others, both authors and readers, become more literate in Critical Caritas-Veritas Literacy Consciousness as a way of being and becoming for living Caritas-Veritas as the core values foundation of being-becoming—moving beyond the task busy-doing culture, beyond the Caritas-Veritas Illiteracy of institutions and the dominant technical practice models.

The Critical Caritas-Veritas Literate nurse and health practitioner becomes part of a global vision of health and human evolution. Critical Caritas-Veritas Literacy is engaged in service to humanity at a different level by radiating the energetic field of Caritas-Veritas through overt and subtle practices, affecting the entire field. Critical Caritas-Veritas Literate nurses and partners become the Caritas field for unitary caring science praxis, transcending and re-patterning the conventional task illiteracy (Watson 2008).

In being Caritas-Veritas, in living Caritas-Veritas Literacy, we become bodhisattvas in the Buddhist view; that is, we become those who bless others and become blessings to self and others. We become evolved and awake, and we actively affect the entire universal field of humanity (Watson 2008).

Now more than ever, with the current geo-political, social discourse media bordering on violence and even civil and global war, we and the pubic alike are called to lift our consciousness beyond Paradigm I and II thinking. To sustain our moral commitment to human caring, love of humanity, healing, and wholeness, we need discipline-specific, professional reminders of that which we know and knew all along but have lost: our core morality—Veritas values—must continuously evolve for self/other. We need a language to remind us, to capture the truth of moral commitment that sustains nursing's caring-healing service to humanity across time. Caritas and Veritas are virtues framing the moral foundation of our profession; they are and have been unmovable, enduring, stable, and timeless. Here I bring them forth through this language as a way to keep alive our shared humanity and values across time.

Unless nursing continues to evolve in its unitary awakening and moral literacy as the foundation of a distinct discipline, there is little to no hope for survival of the discipline as a field of study and practice. Unless we continue to explore the nursing phenomenon within its own paradigm, it will not be fulfilling its scientific, ethical, professional covenant with its public or itself. Indeed, if nursing does not attend to its disciplinary knowledge-practice development, which includes a rich moral, philosophical, caring values commitment, perhaps it should not exist.

Concepts of Caritas-Veritas Literacy offer a new emphasis in Unitary Caring Science as an area of disciplinary, philosophical-ethical inquiry. This focus relates back to structural elements of Unitary Science and a unitary view of axiology, the philosophical study of values and morality. It is an invitation for scholars in nursing and related disciplines to explore the disciplinary-specific moral values structure in the context of a philosophy of Unitary Science and Unitary Caring Science.

For example, when the phenomenon of Unitary Caring is placed within a model of science,

- Does one's view of science change?
- If so, how does one's view of science change? Does it expand?

- Does caring in science imply or require an ethical, moral philosophical values component for its structure and advancement?
- Does Unitary Science require an ethical moral value component?
- Is Unitary Science somewhat value-free?
- Is unitary science similar to or different from mainstream science with respect to human caring, relationships, meaning, and so on? If so, how?
- Does Unitary Caring Science Praxis require a level of Caritas-Veritas Literacy with respect to values and moral commitment?

It is hoped that these questions will serve as an invitation to additional theorizing, philosophizing, and ethical-empirical knowledge development at the disciplinary and clinical level of Unitary Caring Science Praxis.

CHAPTER SIX

Presence

Caritas-Veritas Literacy

This chapter follows up on the material in chapter 5, which translates presence as a core concept of Caritas-Veritas Literacy. It explores the elusive and transpersonal nature of presence, capturing some of the ways it is treated in the literature and focusing on an expanding view. Caring science is used as a context to integrate and expand some of the core views of presence in the literature. The notion of *Caritas Presence* is introduced as a form of Caritas-Veritas Literacy, conveying a contemporary unitary view of authentic presence with examples.

Presence: An Elusive and Spirit-Filled Concept and Practice

The concept of presence encompasses many life stories and meanings. It is often devoid of facts per se, at least as we know them. Human presence, of course, means many things and has been explored, reviewed, and researched in the nursing and psychological literature in different forms.

The question is: How do we grasp and capture the illusive, spiritual essence and experience of authentic presence, particularly within the nursing community? How can presence be a way of being Caritas, a way of enabling faith and hope as a result of presence? Presence in the more fully developed view becomes praxis, a living Caritas with results.

My book *Caring Science as Sacred Science* (Watson 2005) can serve as a vessel for exploring the elusive experiential, existential-spiritual phenomenon of presence. This view of sacred science acknowledges that a human-to-human connection in a given moment opens and connects with the infinite source of Universal Love energy, creating space for an expanding and evolving consciousness of individuals and humanity. This is transpersonal, beyond ego-physical phenomena, and thus is located within unitary caring science. It goes beyond conventional physical, material objective foci. The unitary caring science model embraces human caring, evolving consciousness, love, and intentionality; Caritas Healing praxis becomes an informed way of living energetic, relational, and spiritual phenomena. Thus, authentic presence requires a unitary awareness that lies beyond the strictly physical presence.

From this point of view, presence can be known only between two or more experiencing persons from their inner life world in the moment. Presence cannot be known from the outside in but only from the inside out, from the subjective life experiences of the people in any given moment. Authentic presence in a given moment between persons captures the human-to-human, spirit-to-spirit connection, which is felt experientially but may not be detected by an outside objective observer.

The ephemeral nature of this form of presence is not unknown or mysterious; all of us have experienced true authentic presence with another and internally recognized this presence in connection with another. We have experienced this human-to-human/spirit-to-spirit/heart-to-heart encounter; we also recognize its absence. How, then, do we make sense of this concept of presence in relation to authentic caring relationships in nursing?

To utilize a common starting point, I conducted a Google search of "presence," which yielded this result: "pres-ence" / prezens / (1) The state or fact of existing, occurring, or being present in a place or thing; (2) a person or thing that exists or is present in a place but is not seen. Example: "The monks became aware of a strange presence."

Presence may also refer to contents (1) technology, (2) entertainment, (3) music. A more technical professional definition and description of presence that can be found in nursing literature was captured by Maggie McKivergin and Jean Daubenmire (1994), who identified three levels of presence. These levels are helpful to differentiate a general definition of presence as an authentic, holistic, human caring professional way of being:

1. **Physical presence:** Being there for the other. This involves actual physical body-to-body contact; for example, physical examining, contact, hugging, doing for, engaging in basic care acts.

2. **Psychological presence:** "Being with" the other. This involves mind-to-mind connection and therapeutic use of self. This includes having the conscious intention to be available to another, engaging in a helping relationship, listening, accepting without judgment (Watson 1999, 2011).

3. **Therapeutic presence:** This notion of presence is closely aligned with caring consciousness, mindfulness, intentionality, loving, openness, at-oneness, intuitive connecting, and spirit-to-spirit connecting; and it is associated with the theory of human caring and "transpersonal caring" (Watson 1985, 2008, 2012). For example, within a caring science context, the levels of therapeutic presence defined by McKivergin and Daubenmire can be translated into transpersonal presence (Watson 1999, 2011).

Nursing theorists, scholars, and students have continued to define and explore the deep meanings of authentic human presence. For example, Danielle Linden at Florida Atlantic University studied the philosophical ontology of authentic presence, guided by the theoretical work of Anne Boykin and Savina Schoenhofer (2001). Likewise, Lynne Dunphy and colleagues (2007), also influenced by the philosophical work of Boykin and Schoenhofer (2001), developed a caring model for a nursing curriculum and for advanced practice. Authentic presence is one of the core concepts of this model and is based on an awareness and knowledge of self, that is, intentionally being with another in the fullness of one's own personhood (Dunphy et al. 2007).

Barbara Dossey and colleagues offer definitions of presence in their editions of *Holistic Nursing* (2000, 2005, 2016). One definition is "Presence: a multidimensional state of being available in a situation with the wholeness of one's individual being; the relational style and quality of 'being with,' rather than 'doing to'" (Dossey, Keegan, and Guzzetta 2000, 208). In their 2005 edition, the authors identify these qualities of presence:

- Self-giving in the moment
- Listening to others
- Knowingly participating in a healing experience
- Giving of oneself
- Being with another in a way the other person perceives as full of meaning (Dossey, Keegan, and Guzzetta 2005, 238).

The authors (2005, 239) further define the notion of "graceful presence" as "an embodiment of divine Love, moving with awareness of sacredness of being—a lightness of being; an intentional love-infused presence—unconditional grace-filled; calm and confident aura radiated when a nurse walks into the room; the gentle tone of voice, the loving touch, genuine connection with eye[s], see[s] patient as whole." These expanded views of presence, from physical to divine grace and the sacred, are congruent with a unitary caring science framework for nursing and Caritas-Healing praxis.

JoEllen Koerner's (2011) work also extends the meaning of presence. She introduced the power of one within an energetic field of consciousness, emphasizing *healing presence as the essence of nursing*. Thus, she advanced the meaning of presence to incorporate healing, thus extending the meaning more deeply. This broadened perspective expressed presence as the spiritual dimension of nursing, incorporating quantum energetic consciousness. As such, Koerner drew upon and expanded Watson's (1999) postmodern book, which developed views of non-physical quantum caring and an energetic field of consciousness as an ontology (a way of being). That is, a conscious, intentional energetic presence occurs when we show up authentically as an open unitary system, co-creating a reality with another person in the moment.

This view is consistent with a transpersonal caring moment and transpersonal presence, reminiscent of the earlier definitions of McKivergin and Daubenmire. This work further helps us understand how our presence becomes praxis and underpins Caritas Process 1 and 2, affirming loving-kindness, faith, and hope.

A more universal development of the phenomenon of presence is found in the work of Peter Senge and colleagues in their book *Presence* (Senge et al. 2004). The authors make an intellectual and emotional case for presence as a core concept, in which presence is considered foundational to human processes within organizations and communities. Such notions of presence support the evolution of organizations and communities, helping them evolve to higher levels of learning and awareness and serving as a gateway to creative change for our shared human future. Senge and colleagues are more specific: "We've come to believe that the core capacity needed to access the field of the future is presence. We began to appreciate presence as deep listening, of being open beyond one's pre-conceptions and historical ways of making sense. We came to see the importance of letting go of old identities and the need to control . . . making choices to serve the evolution of life . . . a process of 'letting come,' of consciously participating in a larger field for change" (Senge et al. 2004, 13). Finally, they conclude that "'presence' is related to a larger field for change and can come from many perspectives—from the emerging science of living systems, from the creative arts, from profound organizational change experiences and from direct contact with the generative capacities of nature . . . congruent with all indigenous or native cultures regarding the universe or Mother Earth" (Senge et al. 2004, 14–15).

Caritas-Veritas Presence: A Converging Unitary Caring Science as Sacred Science View

There are some converging themes among the diverse definitions and approaches to the concept of presence. For example, "presence" is related to the full human radiant presence of being. It goes beyond just physically being present; it goes beyond doing and conveys a deep human-to-human awakened heart, a spirit-to-spirit, heart-to-heart connection—an awakened, quivering, emotional, heart-centered, authentic openness to the *now*.

As Dossey and colleagues (2005, 2016) proposed, this deep expanding notion of presence conveys grace and a sense of divine love, a sacredness and lightness of being. This expanded view is consistent with JoEllen Koerner's (2011) energetic quantum presence as it relates to an energetic field of consciousness. It is transpersonal, transcendent, and postmodern; that is, it goes beyond the ordinary, conventional, modern, objective, physical focus on being.

True transpersonal caring within a Caritas Healing praxis presence is sacred; it dwells in the mystery and unknowns of a larger infinite field. It is beyond the ego and biophysical plane of existence and fulfills the five constituent unitary (everything in the universe is unified or connected) field meanings of caring identified by Marlaine Smith (1992a, 14–28): "manifesting intention; appreciating pattern; attuning to dynamic flow; inviting creative emergence; opening to and experiencing the infinite." Thus, an authentic transpersonal unitary caring presence is consistent with the practice of unitary caring science as sacred science (Smith 1992; Watson 1999, 2005, 2008, 2011; Watson and Smith 2002).

A deep human-to-human, spirit-to-spirit presence can be understood as a *transpersonal unitary caring presence,* radiating a new energetic field, which I call the Caritas Field (Watson 2008). Caritas Field conveys transpersonal caring and love and is created between people in the moment, constituting an emergence of a new spirit-to-spirit space within an awakened awareness of oneness (Watson 1985, 2008, 2012).

If we explore presence with this deepening, expansive, converging view, we can consider another level of presence, framed as *Caritas Presence.* This philosophical, theoretical perspective can bring us to an evolved understanding and an enhanced meaning of human caring in nursing and healthcare. This context introduces presence within an expanding and elevated view of human consciousness; new connections can be envisioned among authentic transpersonal caring presence, healing, and the evolution of humanity toward alignment with spirit and Universal Love (Watson 2005, 2008). This level of presence can be considered "biogenic"—life-giving and life-receiving in the moment, "fostering spiritual freedom—restoring well-being [and] human dignity—it is a transforming personal presence that deeply changes one" (Halldorsdottir 1991, 44).

In perennial philosophy and wisdom traditions, presence is associated with "inner presence," which relates to primordial space or egoless-ness (Shambhala Training Glossary 2011); the practice is to empty out, regard other people as yourself, and hold a generosity of spirit toward self and others. One holds this awareness and intentional consciousness of shared oneness toward others without judging or placing them in a particular mind-set. It is "mind without fixation" (Shambhala Training Glossary 2011, 3).

Caritas Presence as praxis involves a discipline of "standing still," holding that heart-centered loving-kindness inside while open and available. One is open to give and receive all that is spontaneously arising in the moment—free of ego attachment—allowing for creative emergence in the now.

Caritas Presence as praxis is manifest by these processes, rituals, and intentional acts (Watson and Browning 2012):

- Begin with centering—preparing for a caring moment.

- Practice pausing, silencing, "emptying out" before entering a patient's room, connecting with an inner still point—breathing and releasing from heart-centered stillness, bringing to heart and mind feelings of caring, loving-kindness, and compassion, thus setting one's intentionality and consciousness.

- Radiate this heart-centered gratitude of loving-kindness and compassion for self and other.

- The goals of radiating beyond self are to open to the unitary field of universal source for alignment, to manifest a caring-healing environment, to "be/become" an energetic healing environment for self and others, manifesting a Caritas Field.

- The patient's family experiences the calming, soothing energetic field of Caritas Presence—that is, an authentic heart-to-heart, spirit-to-spirit connection of loving-kindness and compassion. This level of Caritas Presence transcends the presenting situation, whereby both patient and nurse experience an authentic caring moment connection. Caritas Presence opens to a new field of consciousness of new possibilities. Both nurse and patient can share Caritas spirit-to-spirit consciousness, opening access to the universal energy of infinite love.

This level of presence may be beyond conventional views of presence in the literature. Caritas Presence is transpersonal, beyond ego and physical dimensions. Caritas Presence touches the sacred life force of self and others, honoring the unitary life force. However, it is becoming increasingly evident in theory-guided practices of human caring in clinical settings.

Examples of Caritas Presence as praxis include ethical-spiritual ways of being with another. They include such personal/professional practices as:

- Loving-kindness and equanimity
- Deep attentive silent listening
- Awakened heart-centered feelings
- Compassionate forgiveness
- Gratitude and deep appreciation
- Giving–receiving
- Stillness–silence
- Open to the power of one, the infinite field of Universal Love/source
- Manifest/radiate a caring-healing energetic loving field beyond self.

These notions of Caritas Presence (Watson 2008) as praxis are already known at some level; we bear witness to self-other when we hold a caring consciousness and intentionality of love or compassionate presence toward another in a given moment. One's caring consciousness presence in a given moment affects the entire field experience for self and others. In doing so we open our hearts and minds to a sacred space where we can simply be with another, the often unseen process of deep human caring in nursing. This approach to presence captures the essence of our shared humanity, breathing new life into nursing and nurses. We exhale, breathe out, and release the outdated worldview of our separate being and open to our connectedness with all (Koerner 2011; Watson 2012):

Being present requires being authentically oneself, not a role model or a professional façade with distant clinical preconceived judgments and impressions. It requires staying in the other's frame of reference with active attentive listening, without judging. It requires hearing the message and voice of other—hearing the tone behind the words, listening to and seeing the body language; [it] requires listening to the inner voice of one's own intuition. This skill requires recognizing the patient's life story and its meaning to the person, realizing that listening to a patient's story may be the greatest healing gift we can offer. (Watson, cited in Frampton and Charmel 2009, 13)

Within the context of transpersonal human caring theory, Caritas Presence creates a transpersonal caring moment, which in turn can become a healing moment (Watson 1985, 2008, 2009, 2012). This caring moment goes beyond the current moment and becomes part of the larger complex pattern of life and the universe, the infinite field of love that surrounds and encompasses all.

Sacred Presence

Of all the forces
The Strong, the weak,
The gravitational, the electromagnetic
The strangest and strongest force of all
Is the force of LOVE.

ALEX GREY, *ART PSALMS*

In summary, through this shift toward comprehending presence as Caritas-Veritas Literacy as a reverence and sacredness, presence is acknowledged as a part of self, others, and all living things that affect the whole of life. This evolved consciousness reminds us that we all belong to a shared humanity across time and space; we are bound together in this infinite universal field, which holds the totality of life itself (Watson, cited in Frampton and Charmel 2009, 14).

Thus, through Caritas Presence Literacy we learn to be more open, available, and present to the wonders, unknowns, and mysteries of life itself. This expanded, evolved view of presence is consistent with the notion of presence emerging from the science of living systems (Senge et al. 2004); it is located within a global ethic of caring-healing relationships, restoring the sacred in the midst of everyday existence (Watson 2009). Caritas Presence leads us into a larger field and guides us toward what is healthy for the whole, thereby affecting us individually and collectively—it is an inward journey that takes us to the heart of an evolved humanity.

The next section reveals how Caritas-Veritas Literate nurses can become ontological artists and architects of the ancient Yin archetype for healing humanity (Watson 1999).

CHAPTER SEVEN

Arts and Humanities as Archetypes for Caring-Veritas Literacy

Nurse as Ontological Artist and Architect

Truth—Beauty—Art—Serenity—Nature
   That is all there is . . . for this, for everything, we are out of tune
. . . the world is too much with us . . . we lay waste our powers.

   WORDSWORTH

When we enter into the artistry of our humanity, we discover the shared connections of our being in the world. We also discover the light of our creativity, and the human spirit radiating between us creates space for healing. Art and beauty unite us in our humanity, across all cultures and time.

Florence Nightingale revealed that beauty is healing. One of her insights was that a patient should have something beautiful to look at every day. Art serves as a way for us to evolve as humans, to appeal to our highest senses, our better angels, so to speak. I remember a patient saying to me, "I am starved for a work of art." I brought an easel with a great work of art into her stark, institutional hospital room to nurture her longing for beauty and art and to allow her to experience some beauty—food for her soul—to contribute to her healing.

Art has a moral Veritas dimension. It can elevate us; if we are restricted and shut down, our expressions, our emotions, our search for and release of the human spirit, our spirit of humanity can be totalized. That is, we become objectified; our hearts turn to "stony hearts," of which Rumi wrote. Art thus has a function in moral shaping, forming, or deforming.

Art as Infinite Spirit

Estranged from beauty none can be
For beauty is infinity.

EMILY DICKINSON

Emmanuel Levinas, whose philosophical work has informed my writing on the ethics of caring science and unitary caring science, wrote about the infinity and the totality of our humanity. Levinas (1969), along with Teilhard de Chardin (1959) and others, such as the twelfth-century Hildegard of Bingen, explored the reality that there is an infinite evolution for humans, for us to evolve to higher and higher levels of our consciousness and connection with the greatest source of all—the infinite field of Universal Love, the Omega point (Teilhard de Chardin).

In art we see beauty as evolving spirit as well as creative inspirations and expressions; there is no end to our infinite consciousness expansion and creativity for diverse ways of seeing and being in the world, in exploring the wonder and awe of our universe. Without expression of the human spirit revealed through art, beauty, serenity, silence, sound, and nature, we witness the opposite: totalizing. The opposite of the infinite evolution of our humanity is the totalizing of our humanity, whereby we reduce self and others to the moral status of an object. As that happens we can justify restricting human evolution or expressions of emotions, meaning; we justify treating others as objects.

In shutting down our connections and evolution of the whole, we avoid our own being-becoming and restrict life for others, our world. Without this awakening to art and artistry for the survival of humanity and the world, we are faced with rhetorical questions from T. S Eliot: Where is the life we have lost in the living? Where is the wisdom lost in knowledge and information?

Art as Soul Care

The arts open us to unknown experiences and the unlimited diversity of human expressivity, which had been dormant within the human heart and soul. As Ralph Waldo Emerson captured it, the soul seeks beauty. It is one expression of the universe. The Russian artist Wassily Kandinsky described it this way: the spiritual resides in art. Art is an archetype for the soul; art ensouls our world and our universe.

More recently, it was acknowledged that the future of veterans' care is going to be soul care. The wounds veterans carry have to be addressed and healed at the soul level, not just at the body-physical level alone (2015 GetWell Network conference, Washington, DC).

In reality, in an awakening to the human spirit and soul care, we can acknowledge that all true unitary caring—Caritas-Veritas Literacy—is soul care. That is what is missing in our dominant medical systems. That is why art, beauty, nature, color, light, form, taste, and sound have to return to models of Caritas-Veritas Literacy as a guide to Unitary Caring Science Praxis if healing is to be honored beyond body machine care. As Parker Palmer (2004) stated, our ways of knowing can either form or deform the human soul. In the outdated world of dominant medical care, we can and have deformed the human soul. That may be one reason the public is crying out for another way to attend to healing, health, well-being, well-becoming. That is why nursing has such a critical role to play in "ensouling" the healthcare system with new models of caring-healing whereby the artistry of our being is built into consciousness.

Nurse as Ontological Archetype/Artist/Architect

As I outlined in my book *Postmodern Nursing and Beyond* (1999), nurses have been explored as "ontological archetypes," "ontological artists," and "ontological architects." Each of these postmodern and post-postmodern dimensions—archetype, art, and architect—represents the energy of ancient archetypal yin, feminine healing, serving as artist through caring-healing acts. Indeed, Florence Nightingale said that nursing is the finest of the arts: nurses as artists affect the environmental field, which becomes the energetic Caritas-Veritas field (Quinn 1992). In this level of literacy the nurse becomes an ontological architect for creating new ways of being human in the midst of sterile institutional environments. For example, nurses who practice unitary caring science have created healing sanctuaries for self-caring, caring spaces for the artistry of their own expression and creativity—bringing humanity, life, beauty, and serenity back into sterile, busy medical-technical systems.

We see signs of new hospital designs integrating art into what is referred to as "psycho-architecture," even incorporating components of sacred geometry into the new plans. Virginia Commonwealth University Hospital in Richmond, Virginia, has created "Watson Rooms" in every unit of the hospital. One of the CEOs told me that they interviewed architects they were hiring to design a new tower as to whether they knew what "Watson Rooms" were. Only one architect knew what they were; that is the one they hired to build the new tower for the hospital, designed so every unit has a "Watson Room." This momentum is simply an example of the evolving consciousness of the need for beauty, art, serenity, silence, calm, and space in which the souls of practitioners as well as patients/family can "catch up" by experiencing the basic human need for space and quiet. This need is essential for nurses as well as patients/families and every staff member. It is particularly pressing for nurses to have such space so they can pause and center themselves in the midst of their hectic pace.

Simple environmental healing acts that nurses can control, like dimming the lights and having quiet time, become artistic acts of healing for all. Nurses' consciousness and intentionality to practice caring science theory and philosophy create communities of caring at the unit level, practicing Caritas Processes for self and others.

I refer to nurses who possess this consciousness as participating in a "Caritas Conspiracy"—now a Caritas-Veritas Literacy Conspiracy because the higher vibration of caring and love affects the entire unitary field. Taking time out to support each other, to pause and center before entering a patient's room, before conducting business meetings are also acts of caring that become transformative Unitary Caring Literacy art—acts of healing for self and system.

A Native American elder advised me, "Every day we should do an act of power and an act of beauty." Our caring-healing acts, both simple and grand, become acts of beauty and therefore become acts of healing. Art lifts the veil of our feminine energy, uncovering the Caritas-Veritas Literacy—the hidden yin goddess behind the gods in the universe that carry the heavy energy of yang. Art is the healing yin: she who lifts the spirit and lightens the energy; she who nurtures the soul with her expression, kindness, patience, love, caring, compassion, passion, expressivity of unlimited diversity; she who offers understanding, acceptance of all things that are human-divine as one.

No human being can heal with yang energy alone; we need balance of yin with yang energy for healing. Yet our healthcare systems, including many conventional nursing practices, are organized around yang energy. Yin energy, emanating from nursing and all the vicissitudes of art and artistry, contributes to and is needed for healing. Artistry of being is a lifelong search for the beloved, the great source: our creator of the universe. Our souls need beauty to live.

In shamanic culture, illness is understood as loss of the soul. Healing is a journey to retrieve the soul. Art introduces an energetic flow and movement to access the life force/the soul, which may have been "lost" or dormant, totalized by the busy outer world of physical existence.

Another element of Caritas-Veritas Literacy Consciousness is a reminder about art and artist—that they are here to disturb us. Artists help us see, feel, and be in ways unknown and ambiguous; they move with the spirit of life itself. They capture the impermanence of all movement—of breath and of air itself, a rising up and falling away of each moment.

Indeed, some shamanic practices posit that healing requires an altered state of consciousness, reconnecting us with the spirit within or consciousness beyond the busy mind and scripts that totalize us and our humanity, splitting our soul into darkness and eliminating our one universal common bond, which is life force. We need art to disturb us and also to help us re-pattern our alignment with our own soul/ source/truth (Veritas) art; artistry of caring-healing unites us with Angeles Arrien's (1993) wisdom, the universal soul.

Art as Intentional Healing

There are multiple ways of understanding arts as healing. For example, art taps into the human emotional-subjective inner life world. Art both disturbs and evokes unconscious, archetypal energetic connections for human healing experiences. For example, we see art in a variety of ways. In exploring the various facets of art, one can see how healing arts become Caring Arts Literacy. There are several ways art is known for its healing effect, both from art as inner expression and art as an outer reflection of an inner process, which helps a person or a community resolve and reconcile, integrate pain and suffering. Art is a process of ritualizing and sacramentalizing a traumatic event, releasing and restoring balance and realignment, including shamanic processes and soul retrieval.

Art Intended to Directly Heal: Some Common
Ways Art Is Known for Healing

Art can be used for directed healing by using symbols, images, archetypes, myths, and metaphors that calm and center. Art can activate physiological responses through the calming, soothing vibrations of beauty and nature. The Care Channel (www.Healing health.com), which features the special work of Dr. Susan Mazer and Dallas Smith, is one example of such art. Many hospitals that are guided by unitary caring science and whole person, person-centered care now have the Care Channel as a healing modality for patients, families, and staff to access.

Another example of art that is healing, perhaps directly as well as indirectly, is the work of Alex Grey and his famous *Sacred Mirror* series. One of the programs offered at the University of Colorado's (CU) original Center for Human Caring was a Caring and Arts intensive seminar. I invited Alex to present his work as part of that seminar. In addition to the academic seminar, the CU museum on the Boulder campus made arrangements for his entire installation of *Sacred Mirror* to be in the museum for a public opening. We hosted an open reception for the community as an art program. Some members of the public were so inspired by the vibratory nature of the light that radiated from his art that they would go up to one or more of the great pieces and hold their hands out to receive the energy. Another example was a woman in the community who was hospitalized but had previously heard me present using Alex's *Sacred Mirror* work. She called me to ask if I had a copy of one of Alex's slides. She wanted a copy to meditate on during her hospitalization as an energetic source for visualization and inner healing.

Since then (that was in the mid-1980s), Alex Grey's work is available worldwide in all different forms (www.alexgrey.com/art/). He and his work stand as a universal icon for human evolution of spirit, radiating a living field of universal mind as living energy of God's presence. His work is revered as sacred art, as metaphysical art, as transcendental, as spiritual art. He and his wife, Alyson, are beloved and followed as inspired avatars living their life and their art as higher truths for all of humanity.

Art Created by Artists to Facilitate Their Own Healing

Examples include autobiographical art and representational art depicting incidences of treatment, illness, and change.

My colleague and friend Dr. Mary Rockwood Lane, a faculty associate at the Watson Caring Science Institute, is an example of an artist who created art to facilitate her healing. Her healing art book (Samuels and Rockwood Lane 2013) uncovers how deeply one can heal personally by engaging in art. Mary shares her auto-artistic, autobiographical journey into and out of deep depression after a life-changing personal situation. In her despair she began to paint and literally painted herself back into herself—she healed herself through her own art journey. You can find more information about Dr. Lane on her website and in her books (www.maryrockwood lane.com; www.healingwiththearts.com).

Art That Deals with Specific Aspects of the Healing Process

Pain, loss, changes in body image, grief, and death, as well as hope, change, joy, insights, and so forth, are examples of issues that can be addressed through art. The major art projects during the height of the AIDS crisis are examples of a communal healing process, as is the art that emerged from women with breast cancer who expressed their body image changes and an inner-outer process to bring about integration of the loss and change. These are examples of art that address special aspects of healing, both personally and as a community. This is art that allows the release and return of the human spirit, inviting the soul back into one's body; such diverse opportunities for art following major life trauma, tragedies, war, and famine become critical healing arts for society and for humanity itself.

Recent public marches for peace, Black Lives Matter, and the Women's March on Washington (2016, 2017) are examples of diverse and creative messages of solidarity, of issues affecting human beings.

These are current living examples of communal acts that are forms of communal art to express and reveal the human spirit, the depth of human emotions, of inner longing to advance the human condition, the living field of shared human existence.

Another institutional example of communal art is an experience reported by a psychiatric nurse. She worked in a conventional, chronic, locked ward, where chronically depressed patients existed in a closed setting—an institutional, sterile, gray, lifeless environment with dark paint on the walls. Most of the patients were lifeless, medicated, and immobile.

She had what I would now call Caritas-Veritas Literacy. She created what I call an "Ontological Design" project; she was an ontological artist, but she became an ontological architect.

Here is what she did: she brought in large, wide strips of butcher paper and pasted them all over the walls of the unit. She put out colored markers and crayons openly available for even the most withdrawn patients.

What happened was remarkable: the backward, withdrawn, closed-down, dispirited patients came out from behind the corners of the ward, out from the recesses of the living dead, and began to express and release their inner spirit. They began to mark up the butcher paper with colors, messages, hearts, all sorts of colors, shapes, and designs. I wish I had a copy of the slide that showed the images, designs, colors, shapes, and forms that expressed their artistry of being, radiating new life and human spirit back into the closed, shut-down ward. (I wish I had the name of the nurse who presented this case in October 2011 at the Watson Caring Science Institute, International Caritas Consortium, held in Houston, Texas, sponsored by Michael E. DeBakey, Houston Veterans' Administration [VA] Medical Center.) She was a nurse at the Houston VA, demonstrating evidence of Caritas-Veritas Literacy as an example of Unitary Caring Science Praxis. She may be surprised to realize that this was what she was really doing/being, even though she thought of it as a creative psychiatric nursing practice.

This was a spontaneous art act of a nurse, demonstrating and freeing the human spirit.

This example reminds me of R. D. Laing's message about psychiatric emergencies. I heard him speak in a seminar in Boulder, Colorado, many years ago. He said a psychiatric emergence represents an "emergence of the spirit." This one simple art act serves as an exemplar of a nurse literate in Caritas-Veritas who was allowing for the emergence of spirit as an ontological artist and likewise an ontological architect. This act of human artistry also reveals and reflects the sacred feminine energy of nurse as archetype, needed to balance and complement the otherwise sterile, dehumanized, soulless medical-technical system.

> My soul's reverence for creation increases every time
> I behold the miracle of a sunset or the beauty of
> The Moon.
>
> MAHATMA GANDHI

Artist-Designed Psycho-Architecture; Healing Spaces/Healing Architecture

This type of art/architecture makes a conscious, intentional, even a technical, precise scientific effort to integrate symbol, myth, archetype, mystery, and legend into architectural and environmental themes. Such art can be considered "ontological design," an integration of sacred geometry into architectural structures so that humans can "be" and feel differently. As the healing architecture field evolves, I predict that future hospital architecture will systematically incorporate a sacred geometry environment, energetically and aesthetically contributing to healing experiences.

Healing Arts as Discipline-Specific Caritas-Veritas Healing Practice

When we go deeper into art and healing, as we find a release of human spirit and creativity, we uncover universals of healing. Drawing on the work of Angeles Arrien (1993), an anthropologist and wisdom teacher of ancient indigenous cultures worldwide, several universal questions can be addressed as forms for healing arts, healing the human spirit or loss of soul. These areas are also shamanic teachings. The questions asked of a sick person are:

- When did you stop singing?
- When did you stop dancing?
- When did you stop being enchanted by story? (myth? symbols? metaphors? images?)
- When did you stop receiving comfort?
- When did you stop experiencing the sweet solace of silence? Spirit of nature?

Any one of these haunting questions reflects the fact that the ill person is dispirited—separated from his or her soul/source. This, too, reminds us of illness reflecting the loss of soul or separation from the soul. The arts in any form help any of us in any culture to recover our soul/our spirit, which is calling us to come back into right relation with who we truly are in spirit—purity of Veritas, of being-becoming.

These lingering questions can be addressed through nursing and unitary caring science. Once we step into unitary caring science and we have the literacy of Caritas-Veritas as our moral guide to praxis, there is an unlimited, infinite variety of arts/artistry/creativity, both formally and informally, that we can draw upon, even in a given moment. Even our movement with a patient can be healing; our touch, our presence, our love—each of these can be uncovered in infinite ways of artistry, of being human. Through using arts as intentional forms and through simple artistic acts of human caring, the Caritas-Veritas Literate nurse more consciously and intentionally serves as archetype, artist, and architect for the release of human spirit and for introducing and sustaining artistry as a way of being human.

Caring-Healing Arts as a Guide to Unitary Caring Science Praxis
Taking the arts to another level, we can translate the literacy of Caritas-Veritas Artistry into a manifestation of Unitary Caring

Science Praxis. By understanding the arts as a manifestation of praxis, we incorporate the artistry of humanity into our discipline-specific practices; the healing arts reflect caring values (Veritas), our artistry of being human, consciousness (Caritas), and our awareness of the human need to express the fullness of humanity in diverse and infinite ways (unitary). This area incorporates the entire range of energetic caring-healing modalities and encompasses the practice of the ten Caritas Processes. This growing area intersects with developments in complementary-integrative medicine-nursing and mind-body medicine, energy medicine.

The Caring-Healing arts open us to the entire unitary healing field, acknowledging the phenomenon of non-local consciousness and offering new explanatory models—for example, prayer, meditation, the placebo effect of human caring relations, spiritual healing, distant healing, spontaneous remission, miracles, mystery. These arts affirm the role of love, relationships, purpose, meaning, connections, support, faith, hope, consciousness, silence, and intentionality in a healing environment. They incorporate the range of contemporary and ancient East-West techniques, such as acupressure, acupuncture, Tai Chi, healing touch (HT), therapeutic touch (TT), tender touch, and intentional touch, including music-sound, art as soothing and calming, and sounds of nature. All of these modalities and approaches to treatment and healing can be understood as discipline-congruent with the nursing Caring-Healing Arts.

Healing Art Intersects with the Ten Caritas Processes® as Healing Art/Acts

The ten Caritas Processes® as healing arts incorporate yet transcend medical treatment and patient outcomes. Florence Nightingale's *Notes on Nursing* (1969) serves as a historic nursing blueprint for nursing caring acts as arts—redefined under unitary caring science as caring-healing modalities while acknowledging that Caritas Processes become a healing art in themselves. More specifically,

Nightingale noted modalities for health that can be classified as auditory, visual, sensory, olfactory, consciousness, tactile dimensions of basic care, including color, light, nature, form, position of the bed, sound, noise, and voice. All of these areas can be directly translated into healing arts energetic modalities—for example, music, sound, art, touch, aromatherapy, room color, reflexology, light, and psycho-architecture, including more recently the healing environment. (See Watson 1999, 2011, for more on the healing environment. Also see www.HealingHealth.com. The popular hospital-based Care Channel, developed by Dr. Susan Mazer and Dallas Smith, serves as a contemporary example of systems purposefully creating a healing arts environment.)

Unitary caring science seeks to combine science with the humanities and the arts. Unitary caring science thinking is not neutral with respect to human values, goals, subjective individual perceptions, and meanings. It is not detached from human emotions and their diverse expressions, be they culturally bound or individually revealed. Caring science is not separate from human spirit, the physical/metaphysical/spiritual lattice of universal oneness.

The discipline of nursing—guided by a unitary caring science orientation—seeks to study, research, explore, identify, describe, express, and question the relation and intersection between and among the ethical, ontological, epistemological, methodological, pedagogical, and aesthetic—*honoring all ways of being and becoming more human, more humane.*

These art/aesthetic caring-healing modalities can be framed as a form of Caritas-Veritas Literacy for healing as a means toward a mature nursing praxis. Manifestations of praxis in action can alter, if not transform, nursing practices, healthcare policies, and administrative decisions.

CHAPTER EIGHT

Integrative Nursing*

Unitary Healing Principles

The arts and humanities have been positioned within a Unitary Caring Science praxis as a mode of living Caritas-Veritas Literacy. The previous chapters offered an explication of the healing arts and unitary paradigm. However, there is a parallel intersection of universal principles of healing and the healing arts with universal principles of caring, developed in the field of integrative nursing.

This focus on integrative nursing is based on the scholarship and programs at the University of Minnesota's Center for Spirituality and Healing, headed by the leadership, scholarship, and research of Dr. Mary Jo Kreitzer. This scholarship is enhanced through the Integrative Fellowship Program at the University of Arizona, Tucson, under the leadership of Dr. Mary Koithan (Kreitzer and Koithan 2014).

---

* This chapter is reprinted/adapted, with permission, from sections of Watson (in press).

This chapter highlights the convergence of the universal principles of caring—à la ten Caritas Processes (Watson 2008, 2012)—with universals of healing, identified as six Integrative Healing Principles (Kreitzer and Koithan 2014). In explicating this convergence we see how clinical Integrative Healing Practices intersect with unitary caring science, relocating healing and the healing arts into an evolved unitary paradigm.

"Integrative nursing is defined as a way of Being-Knowing-Doing [Becoming] that advances the health and wellbeing of persons, families, and communities through caring-healing relationships" (Kreitzer 2015, 1). Kreitzer described integrative nursing as a "framework for providing whole person/whole system care, that is [caring] relationship-based and person-centered and focusing on improving health and well-being of caregivers as well as those they serve" (Kreitzer 2015, 1). Integrative nursing is based on a set of healing principles that are aligned and consistent with Caring Science, as well as on extant unitary nursing theories, including those of Margaret Newman (1999), Rosemarie Parse (1999), and Martha Rogers (1970; Kreitzer 2015). Thus the principles of integrative nursing can be viewed as extant meta-theoretical perspectives that converge under an evolving unitary model and an evolving unitary cosmology of human-environmental oneness.

The following list identifies what can be considered universal integrative nursing principles of human healing. These principles reflect historical values of a unitary, relational, ethical, ontological worldview, including natural inner processes, consistent with Florence Nightingale's view of healing (being in the best possible condition for nature to act). Integrative nursing healing principles incorporate concepts such as wholeness, oneness with nature-universe, infinity, energetic non-physical connections, and innate inner processes and relationships. These integrative nursing principles are consistent with extant unitary nursing theories, unitary science and caring science theory, and a unitary worldview.

Integrative Nursing–Universal Unitary Principles

1. Human beings are whole systems, inseparable from their environment.
2. Human beings have the innate capacity for health and well-being.
3. Nature has healing and restorative properties that contribute to health and well-being.
4. Integrative nursing is person-centered and caring relationship-based.
5. Integrative nursing practice is informed by evidence and uses the full range of therapeutic modalities to support/augment the healing process, moving from least intensive/invasion to more, depending on need and context.
6. Integrative nursing focuses on the health and well-being of caregivers as well as of those they serve. (Keitzer and Koithan 2014, 7–21)

These healing principles reflect a unitary ontological worldview of energetic universal connections and relations. They allow for physical and metaphysical phenomena, objective–inner-subjective human relational experiences, and natural inner healing and health, evolving beyond empirical science physical phenomena of human experiences and beyond medical technical intervention.

Ten Caritas Processes® of Unitary Caring Science

Next, we see how integrative nursing principles of unitary healing (Kreitzer and Koithan 2014) intersect with the ten Caritas Processes of Transpersonal Caring Theory—all consistent with Unitary Caring Science. Unitary Caring Science contains the six universal principles of human healing as seen in the core principles of caring: the ten Caritas Processes (Watson 2008, 2012). These combined principles and processes posit human caring and Infinite Love as an ethical, philosophical, ontological guide for the discipline of nursing.

While integrative nursing identifies universal principles of healing, Caritas Processes provide the language for human caring. Without a shared language and a unifying disciplinary ethical, philosophical, ontological foundational structure, nursing's caring-healing practices and principles are unknown and invisible and are rendered nonexistent. By identifying the shared unitary characteristics of integrative nursing (IN) and Unitary Caring Science (UCS), new congruent dimensions are identified.

Shared Disciplinary Characteristics of UCS and IN Provide Premises for Unitary Caring Science Praxis

- UCS-IN praxis principles involve universality of human caring-healing as a unitary phenomenon.
- UCS-IN praxis principles build on the ten Caritas Processes® of Caring Science and transpersonal caring as a theoretical guide for expanding nursing's disciplinary foundation for universal caring-healing healthcare.
- UCS-IN praxis builds on the values, ethics, and unitary ontology of the nursing discipline, informing relational-ethical accountability and ontologically designed caring-healing systems with the infinite global emergence of caring-healing healthy communities.
- UCS-IN praxis builds on universal principles of human healing and Caritas Processes of transpersonal caring.
- Together, UCS-IN creates a universal caring-healing language, exploring evidence of love as an energetic source of healing. (Malloch and Porter-O'Grady 2010; Watson 2008, 2017)
- UCS-IN praxis is guided by the unitary Ethic of Belonging and Love as nursing's discipline-specific, unitary ethical view of science—allowing for concepts such as non-local consciousness, non-physical phenomena, the human caring transpersonal field, human health-healing experiences, mystery, and infinite unknowns.
- UCS-IN praxis grounds the discipline within an expanding unitary view of science, adhering to nursing's moral-ethical imper-

ative as the starting point to sustain humanity itself and specifically human caring-healing and health practices for our world.

- UCS-IN praxis offers directions for whole person–whole system, caring-healing, global healthcare organizations.

Summary

Caring Science, Unitary Caring Science, and integrative nursing have evolved both in parallel and separately. However, by using a disciplinary ontological-ethical matrix analysis, convergence and synergy can be uncovered between Caring Science and integrative nursing, contributing to a more comprehensive focus toward a professional praxis model for deep caring-healing healthcare. Unitary Caring Science Principles embedded in Caritas Processes intersect with Integrative Healing Principles, which are considered universals of healing; together, they provide an evolving Unitary Science professional practice model consistent with extant unitary transformative paradigm thinking in nursing.

Contemporary nursing discourse guides provocative new challenges for both integrative nursing and unitary caring science; the challenge is to engage in discipline-specific, unitary knowledge development as the guide to a more mature, evolving, professional, theory-guided moral practice/praxis. As noted earlier, prominent nursing leaders underscore the importance of the discipline of nursing having a shared ontological, philosophical, and ethical foundation. Indeed, without a shared disciplinary worldview, nursing's survivability is at stake (Grace et al. 2016; Barrett 2017; Phillips 2017).

This chapter highlighted how both Caritas Processes and, now, Unitary Caring Science and integrative nursing healing principles adhere to extant unitary nursing ethical, ontological, paradigmatic, and philosophical worldviews. By exploring and uncovering shared disciplinary characteristics of IN and UCS, a new synthesis emerges for a higher-order, comprehensive professional praxis model.

Conclusion

New healthcare caring-healing models will be required to participate in a unitary world beyond restrictive medical treatment and cure models. Nursing's commitment to sustain humanity calls for advanced models of professional caring-healing and health. It invites new provocative thinking and critique if nursing is to evolve and serve a new world of global health for all. Together, unitary human caring processes and human healing offer a new unitary, discipline-specific model to underpin nursing praxis. Without the language and clarity of a discipline-specific framework of caring-healing for nursing, the nursing profession becomes marginalized, institutionalized, and thwarted. A Unitary Caring healing framework that binds together universal principles of human caring with universal principles of human healing not only helps advance nursing's timeless professional ethos; it also helps in actualizing nursing as a distinct health discipline in service to global humanity.

Living Examples of Caritas Praxis in the Field

From Clinical Agencies and Sites in the USA and Other Countries

This section includes living exemplars of discipline specific, theory-guided practice models of Caring Science. Each inclusion reflects a visual representation of Watson's human caring-healing philosophy and Caritas Process-es. Several of the representations in the United States are from designated National Caring Science Systems of the Watson Caring Science Institute or living examples of implementing caring theory in their setting.

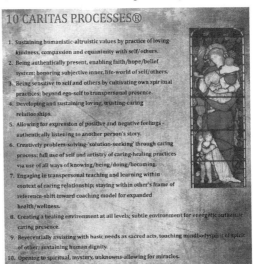

10 CARITAS PROCESSES®

1. Sustaining humanistic-altruistic values by practice of loving-kindness, compassion and equanimity with self/others.
2. Being authentically present, enabling faith/hope/belief system; honoring subjective inner, life-world of self/others.
3. Being sensitive to self and others by cultivating own spiritual practices; beyond ego-self to transpersonal presence.
4. Developing and sustaining loving, trusting-caring relationships.
5. Allowing for expression of positive and negative feelings – authentically listening to another person's story.
6. Creatively problem-solving-'solution-seeking' through caring process; full use of self and artistry of caring-healing practices via use of all ways of knowing/being/doing/becoming.
7. Engaging in transpersonal teaching and learning within context of caring relationship; staying within other's frame of reference-shift toward coaching model for expanded health/wellness.
8. Creating a healing environment at all levels; subtle environment for energetic authentic caring presence.
9. Reverentially assisting with basic needs as sacred acts, touching mindbodyspirit of spirit of other; sustaining human dignity.
10. Opening to spiritual, mystery, unknowns-allowing for miracles.

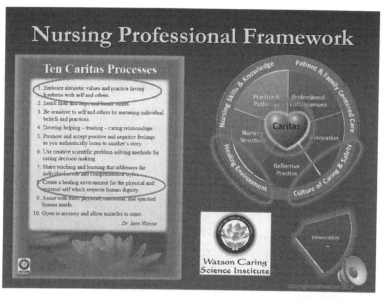

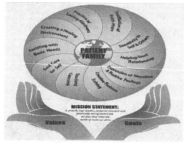

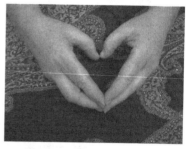

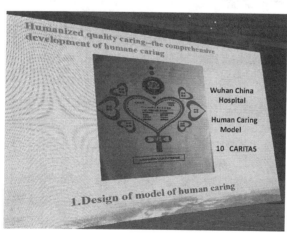

Caritas means "to cherish," St. Joseph's Hospital, Orange, California— courtesy Vivian Norman, Caritas Coach

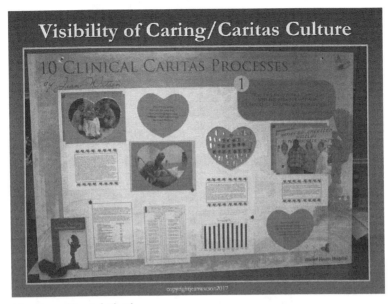

Winterhaven Hospital, Florida

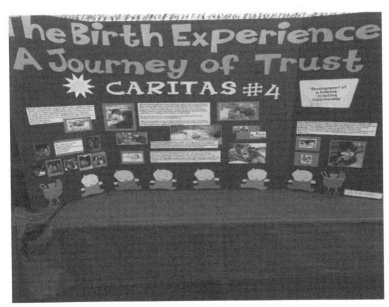

Chilton Hospital, Atlantic Health, New Jersey—courtesy Marcela Klepacki

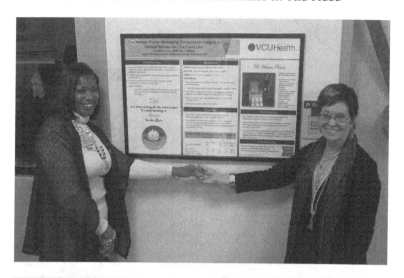

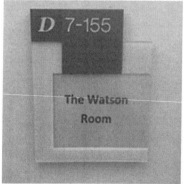
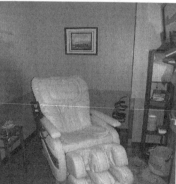

Virginia Commonwealth University Hospital in Richmond, Virginia—courtesy Dr. Crystal Crewe

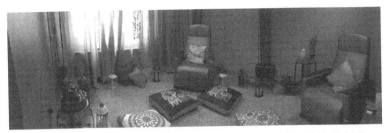

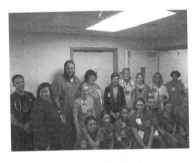

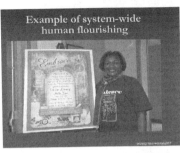

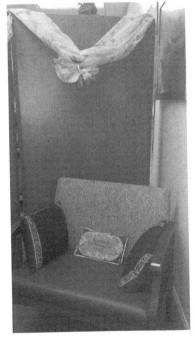

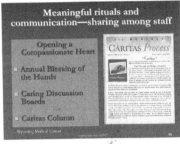

Chilton Medical Center, New Jersey—courtesy Halina Miller

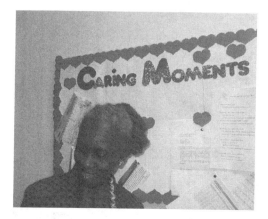
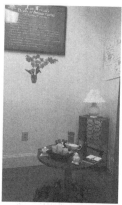

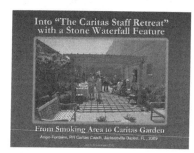
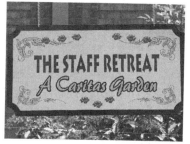

The staff retreat: A Caritas garden, Jacksonville Baptist Health, Florida—courtesy Angie Fontaine

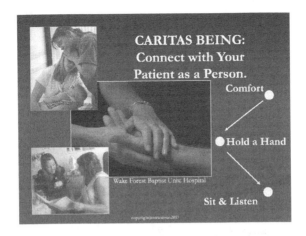

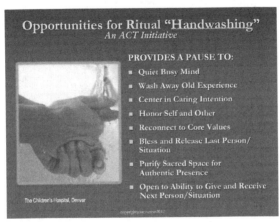

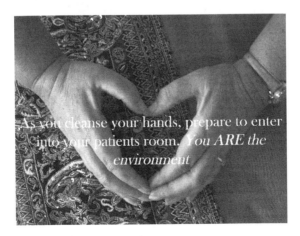

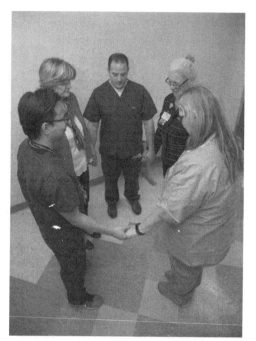

"Holding Circle," St. John Hospital and Medical
Center—Detroit, Michigan

Carl Jung, a Swiss psychiatrist, explains that creating a
circle brings the consciousness of the person or the group
of people toward a center space—a space where insight
and meaning reside. At St. John Hospital and Medical
Center, holding circle is a powerful ritual that bonds us
through the heart and creates space for stillness, accessing
our inner wisdom and intention setting, allowing healing
to occur. It connects us to what the ministry of heal-
ing nursing is called to do. We hold circle at meetings,
conferences, and workshops. We also offer healing circles
for patients and colleagues. Coming together in circle, we
pause, creating space for silences and reflection, and it
allows for the mystery of the unknown to unfold.

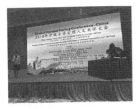

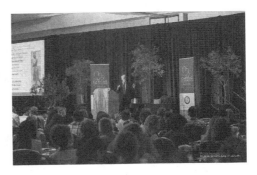

*Kaiser Permanente Northern
California Caritas Consortium. Jim D'Alfonso, leader*

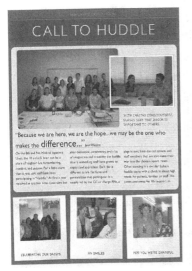

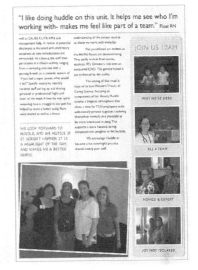

*Children's Hospital Colorado, Aurora, Colorado—courtesy Christine Giffins,
Caritas Coach*

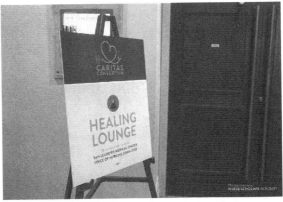

Healing Lounge at 6th Annual Caritas Consortium, May 2007

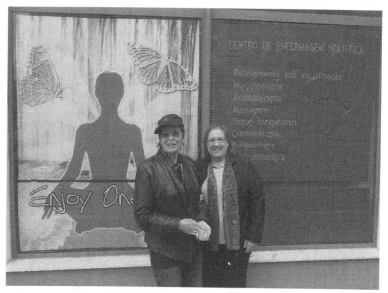

Holistic Nursing Clinic, Braga, Portugal—courtesy Helene Martins

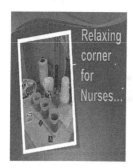

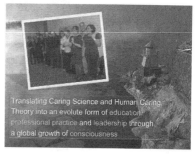

Caring in Progress, Torino, Italy—courtesy Sandra Vacchi

Caring in Progress group, Torino, Italy

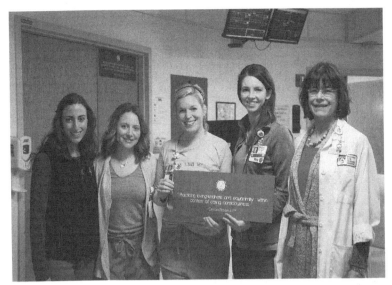

Intermediate neurology unit, Brigham Women's Hospital, Boston. Mary Pennington (nurse director) and Katie Fionte (clinical nurse), at the far right, are Caritas Coaches. Katie's project was to place the Caritas Processes above each patient's door.

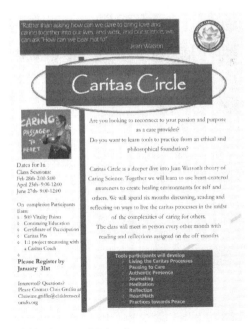

Children's Hospital Colorado

Watson's theory added to the RN self-evaluation tool

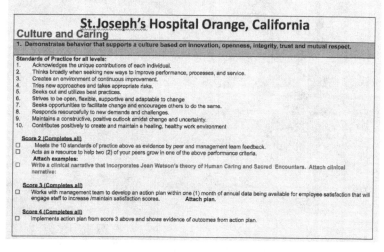

St.Joseph's Hospital Orange, California

Culture and Caring

1. Demonstrates behavior that supports a culture based on innovation, openness, integrity, trust and mutual respect.

Standards of Practice for all levels:
1. Acknowledges the unique contributions of each individual.
2. Thinks broadly when seeking new ways to improve performance, processes, and service.
3. Creates an environment of continuous improvement.
4. Tries new approaches and takes appropriate risks.
5. Seeks out and utilizes best practices.
6. Strives to be open, flexible, supportive and adaptable to change
7. Seeks opportunities to facilitate change and encourages others to do the same.
8. Responds resourcefully to new demands and challenges.
9. Maintains a constructive, positive outlook amidst change and uncertainty.
10. Contributes positively to create and maintain a healing, healthy work environment

Score 2 (Completes all)
- ☐ Meets the 10 standards of practice above as evidence by peer and management team feedback.
- ☐ Acts as a resource to help two (2) of your peers grow in one of the above performance criteria.
  Attach examples:
- ☐ Write a clinical narrative that incorporates Jean Watson's theory of Human Caring and Sacred Encounters. Attach clinical narrative:

Score 3 (Completes all)
- ☐ Works with management team to develop an action plan within one (1) month of annual data being available for employee satisfaction that will engage staff to increase /maintain satisfaction scores.   **Attach plan.**

Score 4 (Completes all)
- ☐ Implements action plan from score 3 above and shows evidence of outcomes from action plan.

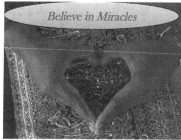

Believe in Miracles

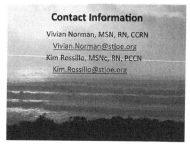

Contact Information

Vivian Norman, MSN, RN, CCRN
Vivian.Norman@stjoe.org
Kim Rossillo, MSNc, RN, PCCN
Kim.Rossillo@stjoe.org

St. Joseph's Hospital, Orange, California—courtesy Vivian Norman and Kim Rosilla, Caritas Coaches

Part Three

CHAPTER NINE

Caritas-Veritas

Toward Unitary Caring Science Praxis

The use of the formalized clinical language of nursing's past preoccupation has lost the capacity for beauty, grace, for evocative metaphors, dreams, inspiration, hope, imagination, creativity, artistry, for
evoking the human spirit. The use of nonclinical language vibrates
at a different level, at a higher frequency than clinical-technical,
sterile words. Thus, we are stretched to consider new depths of
meaning, new experiences and insights, new relationships with the
experiences and the humans we encounter. Nonclinical language
invites and takes us into words and worlds conventional languages
cannot convey. Thus, we need words that are not "fixed," to avoid
words that cannot convey higher vibrations of our humanity and
the universality of our human spirit.

(WATSON 2008, 49)

The next step is to more fully locate Caritas-Veritas Literacy and
transpersonal consciousness within Unitary Caring Science; one
way to do this is through more evocative language, offering a one-

word energetic shortcut for each of the Caritas Processes. This extension into the unitary field leads to a living, active Caritas-Veritas Literacy to inform/transform praxis through an intentional, morally informed Unitary Caring Science.

The one-word terms used to capture the unitary essence and notion of Veritas Literacy underpinning each of the Caritas Processes are from Watson Caring Science Institute Reflective Caritas Cards (Watson and Hope 2011).

The living essence of each Caritas Process practice is captured energetically through the high-value meaning and vibration associated with each word. This essence of Caritas-Veritas vibration connects to a higher vibration of a unitary field. Here we can visualize and energetically grasp the difference between the lower vibration of carative factors (Paradigm I) and the more fluid language of Caritas Paradigms II and III.

The next paragraph and the following section identify one word to capture each Caritas Process. Each process is now embedded as a moral value component of Caritas-Veritas Literacy. This shift locates Caritas Processes more explicitly within the Unitary Caring Science field; it introduces evocative language to capture the essence of Caritas-Veritas Literacy. This unitary field linguistic shift is energetically evocative, tapping into an unconscious association with the meaning behind each Caritas Process. Each word gracefully invites us into Caritas Processes and transpersonal consciousness as a guide to Unitary Caring Science Praxis.

What follows is an invitation into a simple literary language, capturing the instant gestalt of the meaning of Caritas-Veritas Literacy. Each of the original Caritas Processes is captured through one simple word, as follows, and each word, as well as its association with a Caritas Process, is included in chapter 10:

1. Embrace
2. Inspire
3. Trust

4. Nurture
5. Forgive
6. Deepen
7. Balance
8. Co-create
9. Minister
10. Open

Let us fall in love again
And scatter gold dust all over the world.
Let us become a new Spring
And feel the breeze drift in the heaven's scent.
Let us dress the earth in green,
Let the grace from within sustain us.
Let us carve gems out of our stony hearts
And let them light our path of Love.
The glance of love is crystal clear
And we are blessed by its light.

RUMI

While many in the nursing field have studied or are practicing Watson's theory and philosophy of human caring/transpersonal caring, they are not always well acquainted with the universal ten Caritas Processes.

Preparing for any worthwhile endeavor requires the cultivation of values, consciousness, and informed moral skills to engage in doing/being the chosen service to humankind. One cannot enter into and sustain Caritas-Veritas Practices for caring-healing without evolving in his or her consciousness. It is ironic that nursing education and practice require so much knowledge and skill to *do* the job, with focused concentration on technological competencies, but very little effort is directed toward developing ontological competencies/Caritas Literacy skills on how to *be/become*. Nurses often become dispirited, worn down by trying to always care, give, and be there for others without attending to the loving care needed for self. Caritas

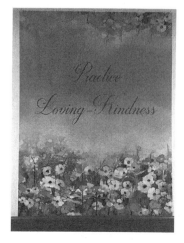

An example of how one system has made visible the practice of loving-kindness, Caritas Process 1, as embraced by nurses in this setting in California. It shows processes of Caritas in action. Other national/international clinical caring science visuals are depicted in other photos in this book. Courtesy, Gloria Littlemouse and Los Alamitos Medical Center, Los Alamitos, California. Used by permission.

invites, if not requires, nurses to attend to self-caring and practices that assist in their own evolution of consciousness for more fulfillment in their lives and their work.

The figure here represents an example of how theory becomes a living practice. It represents a living Caritas, inviting and affirming nurses and other practitioners engaged in the systematic practice of loving-kindness—hence Caritas-Veritas Literacy.

In this way of thinking, nurses can be models and living exemplars by openly embracing what people have not otherwise made visible. However, here we see loving-kindness openly articulating becoming-being-living Caritas-Veritas work that needs to be done for this planet and humanity at this point in human history. We can become part of a global vision of health and human transformation to help purify the biocidic field; the negativity of violence, abuse, war; and the non-caring illiteracy evident in our medical system.

Practices toward developing Caritas-Veritas Literacy can be supported by my website: www.watsoncaringscience.org. There you can find meditations and inspired teachings to assist you. There are many ways to enter into this kind of evolved unitary awareness. It is only one entry into cultivating an intentional Caritas-Veritas Literacy.

CHAPTER TEN

Unitary Paradigm—Caritas-Veritas

Evoking Paradigm III Words

Words matter / language defines reality . . . Any profession that
does not have its own language in this day and age does not exist
. . . much of nursing clinical language is medicalized-institutional
language.

JEAN WATSON

Perhaps the new role for Caritas-Veritas Literacy is to transform the
vision of human health and healing by creating the energetic unitary field of Caritas-Veritas—using language to name and document
the phenomenon of Caritas, making visible that which is otherwise
invisible. It allows language that embraces both the overt and the
subtle, that creates a unitary opening to practices that transmit and
affect the healing field of the whole.

Exploration of and in-depth background on each Caritas Process
can be found in Watson (2008, 2012), as can an overview on my website: www.watsoncaringscience.org.

In Unitary Caring Science Consciousness, all nurses can contribute to this new consciousness any time they choose. They can do this one by one and become part of creating a deeper level of humanity by fundamentally transforming what happens in a given moment, in a given situation, by experimenting with *being the Caritas-Veritas field*. This includes using language that captures a new unitary paradigm for caring and healing.

As noted in my earlier book (2008), this is the truly deep, noble work of nursing; this energetic field of Caritas-Veritas transcends the conventional way of thinking about nursing and invites a new depth of unitary caring and healing as nursing's contribution to society and global health. This shift acknowledges the Unitary Consciousness of moral value theory–Caritas-Veritas Literacy as one gestalt; it represents nursing's unitary disciplinary commitment and compassionate, moral caring-healing service to self and system and society.

The next section uses one word to capture the essence of each Caritas Process. Each word suggests a higher-energetic vibration and a simple entré into unitary Caritas-Veritas Literacy. The following series of simple words frames each of the ten Caritas Processes.

1. Embrace (Loving-Kindness)

CARITAS PROCESS 1: Cultivating the practice of loving-kindness and equanimity toward self and others as foundational to Caritas-Veritas moral value consciousness (underlying Unitary Caring Science Praxis).

In Unitary Caring Science (Caritas-Veritas)—invites transcendence; transpersonal, allowing for consciousness evolution; open to the touching infinity of cosmic-divine love.

2. Inspire (Faith-Hope)

CARITAS PROCESS 2: Being authentically present; enabling faith-hope/belief; honoring the subjective life world of self/other.

In Unitary Caring Science (Caritas-Veritas)—appreciating pattern; authentic sacred presence.

3. Trust (Transpersonal Self)

CARITAS PROCESS 3: Sensitivity to self/others; cultivate one's own spiritual practices—beyond ego to transpersonal presence.

In Unitary Caring Science (Caritas-Veritas)—Inner self/self-love; higher self/source experiencing divine love; spirit; touching infinite cosmic love; movement toward Omega point.

4. Nurture (Relationship)

CARITAS PROCESS 4: Develop and sustain helping, trusting, loving, caring relationships.

In Unitary Caring Science (Caritas-Veritas)—vibrating heart-centered unitary connections; spirit-to-spirit heart connection; attuning to dynamic flow.

5. Forgive (All)

CARITAS PROCESS 5: Allow for expression of positive and negative feelings; authentically listen to another person's story.

In Unitary Caring Science (Caritas-Veritas)—nonjudgmental acceptance; holding sacred space; attuning to dynamic flow; grace.

6. Deepen (Creative Self)

CARITAS PROCESS 6: Creative use of self and all ways of knowing; artistry of Caritas nursing.

In Unitary Caring Science (Caritas-Veritas)—allowing for creative emergence; "reading" the Caritas field; becoming the Caritas field; trusting intuition.

7. Balance (Learning)

CARITAS PROCESS 7: Engage in transpersonal teaching-learning-caring relationships and subjective meaning.

In Unitary Caring Science (Caritas-Veritas)—appreciating pattern; inner listening/learning; wisdom.

8. Co-Create (Caritas Field)

CARITAS PROCESS 8: Create a healing environment at all levels; subtle environment.

In Unitary Caring Science (Caritas-Veritas)—appreciating pattern; re-patterning; radiating energetic heart presence; "being" the Caritas field.

9. Minister (Humanity)

CARITAS PROCESS 9: Reverentially assisting with basic needs as sacred acts; sustaining human dignity.

In Unitary Caring Science (Caritas-Veritas)—Sacred service; manifesting intentions; immanent-transcendent; body-spirit are one.

10. Open (Infinity)

CARITAS PROCESS 10: Open to spiritual, existential, mysterious; allow for miracles.

In Unitary Caring Science (Caritas-Veritas)—experiencing the infinite; transpersonal, pan-dimensional; transcendent; esoteric; ecstatic; distant healing; belonging.

Un-Concluding Postscript Fragments

Metaphysics and Unitary Caring Science

Caring for others takes place, so to speak, in the metaphysical realm. We cannot "see" this realm, but we experience it. Over and over I watched the caregiver and the person accepting care as they came to constitute one wholeness. When two of us enter into each other this way, willingly and receptively, transformation takes place. The gestalt of our separate beings loosens and vibrates. The material of our being and becoming begins to flow. We experience ourselves and each other as elemental substance. We experience the living field of our interconnectedness. And we are filled with energy, a living material, palpable, substantial [energy]. This energy is nearly visible in the air around us. It is as though we give off light.

These moments of transcendence are fascinating. They occurred again and again, each time flowering forth, a moment of intense energy, of very material presence. I felt I was witnessing the invisible made substance. I was witnessing the spirit made flesh.

—FROM KRYSL 1989

This is an epilogue of free association and un-concluding questions or loose thoughts about unitary caring science and how it can take us to new explorations of the infinite field of Universal Cosmic Love (Levinas 1996), to a higher/deeper level—yes, a metaphysical level. Can unitary caring science explore metaphysical phenomena with integrity and authenticity and be scientifically legitimate? Or can we really start with a new beginning for unitary caring science as one that has ethics as its starting point?

In this instance, Emmanuel Levinas's view of "the Ethic of Belonging" (to the infinite field of love) becomes the first principle of unitary caring science and in turn offers a new/old explanatory, non-physical model of caring-healing. This expanded worldview or cosmology accommodates new meanings for phenomena such as non-local consciousness, miracles, mystery, unexplained healings, prayer, distant healing, and other existential-spiritual, mystical unknowns.

Unitary caring science and unitary field views embrace a relational, unitary ontology/worldview; they make it explicit that being human involves relation, connection, and unity with self, others, all living things/Mother Earth/the cosmos. Likewise, unitary caring science and unity of being embrace transcendence, bowing to that which is greater than self, greater than physical existence alone but open to wonder, awe, mystery, miracles, the sacred unknowns, the holy.

A unitary caring science grounds nursing and other health professionals and the public alike; it helps us all find new meanings where there may be a void in meaning; it offers new explanatory models for phenomena Western science cannot handle. Here in Unitary Caring Science, we enter the universal sacred circle of life, honoring and bowing to our connection with a quantum spirit-filled worldview of unity that transcends previous thinking while also embracing it.

This epilogue can serve as a primary disciplinary source for exploring nursing's most evolved paradigm of unitary caring and unitary caring science. It will also help transform and expand the thinking of students, practitioners, scholars, and administrators about human caring-healing phenomena, leading to new unitary models of nursing and healthcare praxis.

Alfred North Whitehead (1985) indicated that all science starts with ontological assumptions. That is, what does it mean "to be?" To be human? What is the ultimate sense of existence?

These domains of discourse now lead us to metaphysics and non-physical phenomena and universal cosmic views of a unitary worldview in which love holds everything together in the universal infinite field. Both science and philosophy have acknowledged that they seek to explore truth. Therefore, in the world of philosophy, theory, and science, we seek a theoretical explanation of phenomena that resonates with a new existential-spiritual truth of the non-physical–physical existential which humanity can acknowledge and proclaim and with which it can engage: "If there is no attempt or even interest in finding patterns that connect the intrinsic basic features that humanity shares, then we are no longer a wildly diverse, radiant, holistic ornament of Spirit; we are shattered fragments of stained glass scattered in a grey and barren landscape . . . destined to cut each other . . . The world, just as it is . . . is a perfect, whole, radiant ornament of Spirit. That is the Absolute nature of everything" (Bigelow 2008, xiv–xv).

Ancient Mayan Teachings: Mayan Calendar

There are five epochs in human history, each lasting approximately 5,000 years.

First was Stone Man, followed by Clay Man, then Wood, followed by Corn Man; and now, since 2012 we are in [the] era of Metal Man. Thus, we are now in a new epoch of human universe evolution. Metal Man is the era whereby the human has greater and greater capacity to communicate globally and virtually. However, the Metal era evolution results in an advanced technological human but without a heart.

The other dimension of the Metal epoch is that humans are now more capable of communicating with other Beings from a non-physical plane and vice versa. For example, there are more and more sightings of those ancient ones from the other side showing up, coming to teach us.

INTERVIEW WITH BENJAMIN, MAYA ANTHROPOL-
OGIST AND EXPERT GUIDE, TULUM AND COBA,
MEXICO, DECEMBER 22, 2016

After my accident, when I had to be quiet for up to three months, I began to have biblical dreams and mystical experiences beyond my usual realm of existence; they were of a higher dimension. They apparently emerged from me being in a contemplative space of stillness and quiet. At one point I was out of body and yet fully embodied.

What was remarkable was experiencing a mystical oneness. I dissolved into total love—I became love. I was not in love or feeling loved or anything else. I just experienced being a constellation of Universal Love. I was love. It felt like a holy experience. In some way, metaphysics and the infinity of love, the awareness of non-local consciousness, help us grasp the fact that we are love. We all come from the sacred universal circle of love, and we all return to love. In our physical, usual, human existence awareness, we forget that we are love.

JEAN WATSON

During my many years of professional travel, I have been priv-ileged to experience and witness the beliefs, patterns, practices, thought systems, and lifestyles of many cultures, religions, and countries around the globe. As recently as this current year, I have been in almost a different country each month; indeed, in some months I was in two and even three countries; during the 2016–17 academic year, I was in eighteen countries. I say this not to glorify the experience but to acknowledge that I have been witnessing and learning from over a million nurses and health professionals for over thirty years.

Without reservation, these experiences have affirmed our human connections and shared beliefs in something that is greater than us, that is beyond our physical existence but exists in the invisible unknown spirit world. While different names are given to the phenomenon, there is a collective knowing that humans seem to share, even though it is in juxtaposition to, or even in conflict with, our daily activities and physical, outer worldview reality world.

Opinions about these metaphysical topics vary widely, since what is being discussed cannot be observed or measured or even truly known to exist.

AUTHOR'S NOTE: The practical implication of definitions of metaphysics and ontology can be translated into programs related to a theory-guided practice of transpersonal caring-healing and the creation of "ontological design" units and systems for hospitals and clinical settings, leading to new ways of being and resulting in new patterns of delivery of caring-healing.

To repeat, the word *metaphysics* has two basic meanings: (1) a branch of philosophy about worldview—for example, the ontology of being; and (2) a branch of philosophy beyond the physical, inviting non-physical reality into our worldview and notions of *being human*. Metaphysics is especially relevant for exploring new explanatory models of non-physical healing, beyond the body physical.

1. Transpersonal Caring—Transpersonal Caring Moment

Transpersonal caring is considered metaphysical in that the entire consciousness of caring and love exists within a single caring moment; that moment transcends time, space, and physicality. Transpersonal also indicates that a new field of connection with infinity is possible in that moment—beyond the ego. There is a spirit-to-spirit connection, opening up space for alignment with source. A transpersonal moment can be a transcendent moment; participants are fully embodied, immanent, and transcendent in the present "now." In Whitehead's view, a transpersonal caring moment is an "eternal now" that holds past/present/future in the one moment: "Transpersonal conveys a concern for the inner life world and subjective meaning of another; however, each are [*sic*] fully embodied, that is embodied in spirit . . . Transpersonal invites a full lovingkindness consciousness [Caritas] in the moment, with an understanding that a transpersonal caring moment can be a turning point in one's life . . . it radiates out beyond the moment, connecting with the universal field of infinity to which we all belong. Thus, the moment lives on" (quoted in Watson 2008, 79).

Transpersonal calls for authenticity of being and becoming a more fully evolved human. This level of existence is at the metaphysical, ethical, ontological level of personal/professional development for health practitioners. This transpersonal consciousness invites spirit and non-physical reality into our daily lives and practices.

Making Meaning from the Starting Point

Taken together, these definitions and combined meanings invite an expanded worldview—acknowledging the non-material universe of energy and spirit while incorporating the material/physical realm of existence. The unitary worldview encompasses views of human consciousness beyond the brain, referred to in the literature as "non-locality of consciousness" (Dossey 1991, 1993; Van Lomel 2011; Alexander 2012); that is, the human physical body resides within a "unitary field of consciousness of all" (Hildegard of Bingen, quoted in Fox 1985). All human beings belong to the "infinite field of Universal Cosmic Love" (Levinas 1996; Watson 2006, 2008, 2012).

In native science and indigenous cultures around the world, people may say, "we all come from the infinite field of Universal Love, and we all return to the infinity of love as the unitary field of everything." Thus, from this metaphysical worldview we can openly honor the sacred circle of life-death as beyond the physical plane of existence, honoring the fact that we are all connected through this field of infinity. Teachings from ancient cultures called this the "active side of infinity" when we allow it to become a part of our entire human-universe field of existence (for example, Castaneda 1998).

Therefore, when we consider metaphysics within these broader meanings, we can invite consciousness, meaning, and purposeful spiritual reflection into our views of what is ultimately existence and what counts as existence. What counts as knowledge? As knowing? As ways of knowing? What does it mean "to be human" on the physical plane? Or are we spiritual beings on the earth plane? These rhetorical questions are bringing new understanding and depth to Teilhard de Chardin's well-known expressed proclamation: *We are spiritual beings having an earthly experience, not the other way around* (Teilhard de Chardin 1925).

This evolved thinking for this time opens up new unitary caring science explorations and new explanations of what can be invited into our life world for transpersonal caring, for healing, even for our understanding of what it means to be: to be human, to evolve, to be whole, to belong. Metaphysics helps us experience transcendence and awaken to our connection with infinity; to participate joyfully in the active side of infinity; to communicate with, invite, and engage in the other realm of existence, often denied or ignored.

With expansion of our minds and hearts into the metaphysics of unitary caring science, we open to the infinite source of cosmic love. Indeed, this discourse invites other spiritual realms of existence to embrace the divine and invites higher frequencies of existence into our physical life field/planet.

Could we then begin to consider spiritual being? Spiritual well-being? Can we consider spiritual healing? Distant spiritual healing? Spiritual intervention? Spiritual surgery? Psychic surgery? Therefore, can we find new explanatory views of phenomena such as miraculous healing? Miracles? Prayer? Unexplainable happenings? Coincidences? Para-psychology? Presence of angels? Ascended masters? Spiritual entities that reside within and beyond the physical plane? Entities that reside within the realm of spirit or in a higher vibratory dimension beyond detection by ordinary senses? These are the provocative questions we invite into our evolving consciousness when we enter into metaphysics in general and the metaphysics of Unitary Caring Science in particular.

Or could we find new metaphysical realities, affirmations, and connections—ethically, philosophically, ontologically, and epistemologically—within Unitary Caring Science for spiritual healing modalities such as Reiki (which draws upon the energy of universal cosmic love)? Healing touch? Therapeutic touch? Intentional touch? Healing presence? Prayer? Caring loving consciousness? Spirit-to-spirit connection in the transpersonal moment? Authentic listening from within? Calling upon spiritual entities? Engaging in spiritual healing interventions?

If we can grasp such phenomena in a new light, within a metaphysical-spiritual context, we can then begin to more fully understand unexplained phenomena of mystical and metaphysical experiences. For example, consider healing phenomena: millions of people from around the world experience healing through St. John of God in Brazil. People in cultures across time have healed through shamanic practices.

Can we trust new understanding and the importance of human experiences as basic as a caring moment—knowing it is transpersonal, which can be a healing moment for all? Metaphysics gives new dimensions to transpersonal caring. Can we deepen our understanding of other non-physical energetic modalities—such as sound healing, aromatherapy, reflexology, acupuncture, acupressure, unlimited still-to-be-identified approaches that help align the physical with the metaphysical/spirit/source/infinite energy of love—to be in right relation with source (universal love), finally acknowledging at many levels that *love is the greatest source of all healing.*

By unraveling definitions and notions of metaphysics, unitary caring science brings the non-physical more prominently into the physical plane for health, healing, and human caring. This book has provided a foundation for a metaphysics of unitary caring science, opening our minds to both an ancient and a contemporary cosmology of "unitary being-belonging-becoming" as moral, ethical, ontological, and epistemological in guiding Unitary Caring Science Praxis; this emerging and constantly evolving worldview underlies the theory of *transpersonal human caring-healing and constantly evolving Caritas-Veritas Literacy to inform praxis.*

Western metaphysics is geared to the static view of reality. "Metaphysics of Unitary Caring Science" unfolds a new era in human history. Can we forgive our history of Western metaphysics? Can Unitary Caring Science move beyond the static views of Western science as we have known it? Can we balance metaphysics as a dynamic starting point and an ongoing process for informing ontology and an evolved epistemology? Can we inspire our science to move us closer to what Teilhard de Chardin identified as the *Omega point*—closer to God consciousness (Teilhard de Chardin 1925), to the universal source of infinity of love? These ways of knowing are what shamans, perennial philosophy, wisdom traditions, ancient teaching, and ancient cultures have proclaimed as truths (Veritas) across time.

This new order of "stepping into metaphysics" overlaps with ethics, ontology, and epistemology to explore the study of truth and to seek theoretical explanations of phenomena that inform praxis-guiding human-caring healing and health.

To address these phenomena scientifically or theoretically, we first have to explore our worldview, our cosmology, our heart's wisdom about science, about truth, about humanity and life itself. These are provocative, spiritual, existential questions for our time and this day and age of *post-truth.* That is, what is the litmus test for truth at this time in our history when we witness distortions of science and data and distortions, if not untruths, presented as new truths, thus underlying the very nature of science and how we understand the meaning of the great circle of life-death.

Western metaphysics has long been obsessed with describing reality as an assembly of static individuals whose dynamic features are taken to be either mere appearances or ontologically secondary and derivative. For Unitary Caring Science, the adventure into the discovery of self/spirit/belonging breaks from traditional metaphysics, which has marginalized, ignored, or avoided them altogether. For example, what is the role of mind in our experience of reality as becoming? What is consciousness outside the physical brain/mind? Are there several varieties of becoming?

Ken Wilber has spent his career exploring these bewildering, if affable, philosophical and scientific adventures and questions, attempting to make sense of them through his writings. For example, he reminds us that "humans are born and begin their evolution through the great spiral of consciousness, moving from archaic, to magic, to mythic, to rational and . . . perhaps into genuinely transpersonal domains. The spiral of existence is a great unending flow, stretching from body to mind to soul to spirit" (Wilber 1996, 35).

How can we understand the emergence of apparently novel conditions? Of unexplained phenomena that clearly exist in human experiences, such as so-called miracles, distant healing, prayer, apparitions of deceased loved ones?

How do we explain the common aspirin? Placebos? The role of the subtle energy of love and touch or even the suggestion of how love changes our body chemistry? How do we explain the effect of such ancient energy practices as Reiki—which is based on accessing universal love as source?

How can we understand the fact that millions upon millions of persons across all epochs of time have sought to communicate with higher levels of existence, even if it is nature itself that is the teacher: learning from the sun-stars, light-dark moon cycles, and elements of earth-air-fire-water; constantly evolving and seeking the meaning of our place in the larger cosmos or universe?

Unitary caring science takes on a double role as both a metaphysical and a meta-philosophical focus for developing a new explanatory model of caring-healing to which millions have already subscribed. While all sciences and philosophies of science aim at the truth, when we step into Unitary Caring Science, we step into metaphysics and a higher/deeper order of truth; further, we seek new forms of epistemology to explore the study of unitary truths that humanity has experienced since time immortal.

Unitary caring science is here on the other side of the infinite field, another reality, yet it is one with the physical plane. Is Unitary Caring Science open to embrace this metaphysical reality, ready to deepen, trust, balance, nurture, co-create our experiences of life and death, living and dying? If so, it is this metaphysical space, when we touch it, that allows miracles, mystery, and unexplained mystical metaphysical phenomena to indeed exist and be validated. Then Unitary Caring Science metaphysics will minister to what millions upon millions of people from around the world have proclaimed across all eras of human history.

As such, our being-becoming-belonging is more whole. We awaken to the wholeness, the oneness of all: one world, one humanity on planet earth, all connected and belonging to one source. Metaphysics opens us to see that ultimately we are one world, one humanity, one heart. When we enter this space of unitary caring, we become peacemakers for our world.

Appendix A

Personal Background
Entrée into Caring Theory / Unitary Caring Science

My original work began as a "treatise on nursing" as an attempt for me to gain more personal meaning from the profession at a time when I was trying to make more sense of nursing and the need for a meaningful philosophical foundation of its science, not merely for it to exist in academe as a subset of medical science. The original work later evolved to serve as a value-guided philosophy, a theory—both middle range and a grand theory to guide our science and our discipline—and an ethic as well as a blueprint for transformative personal/professional life practices.

The original book and efforts in caring philosophy and science "emerged from my quest to bring new meaning and dignity to the work and the world of nursing and patient care" (Watson 1979, 49). When I wrote this book, it was my attempt to find personal meaning in nursing. I was a new faculty member at the University of Colorado, witnessing the rise of academic nursing in a major academic *medical* center campus. I emphasize the word *medical* because that is what it was in the late 1970s and what it remains today, in 2018. Indeed, our campus, which changed its name in the 1980s from medical center to health sciences center, more recently reverted back to its original name but included the named benefactor.

Thus the University of Colorado Anschutz Medical Center (in Aurora) is the current name, setting the imprint for the continuing *medical*-dominated focus on health science to this day. This continues in spite of a vibrant nationally recognized pharmacy school; a nationally ranked dental school; the historically renowned history of the nursing school/college, with a reputation for innovation and leadership; early master's degree programs; and the origin of a nurse practitioner program for the nation and the world. The University of Colorado was also the first public university to offer a clinical doctorate with a focus on caring-healing and health (the nursing doctorate [ND] program), which was preparatory to the national standard degree for nursing practice: the doctorate in nursing practice (DNP).

During my first year in academe, especially after studying philosophy, I felt that our system and even our faculty were somewhat "ignorant," in the sense that they did not know; thus they *ignored* the core foundation of human caring and healing as essential to our profession and the raison d'être and source for survival now and in the future. This is not a criticism; it is a factual comment and commentary on the state of the science and the worldview that continue to drive medical care practices and education to this day. This is also referred to as sick-care approaches to health, caring, and healing. Therefore, my original despair led me to write my first book as a way to find my way home to a meaningful philosophical foundation for nursing science; otherwise, I was thinking that perhaps nursing should not be a part of the university academic medical community if it did not have its own disciplinary foundation for science and practice beyond being a subset of medicine.

However, with a new vision for nursing's future, during the 1980s and into the 1990s the University of Colorado School of Nursing became the leader and the origin of caring science for nursing and health sciences. It was one of the few programs with a PhD focus in caring science, and it created the internationally recognized Denver Nursing Project in Human Caring as well as the Interdisciplinary Center for Human Caring and other prominent health sciences programs.

Thus the early work emerged from my own values, beliefs, perceptions, and experience and my questioning of rhetorical and ineffable issues. For example, what does it mean to be human? What does it mean to care? What does it mean to heal? Questions and views of personhood, life, the sacred circle of the birth-life-death cycle. (My first publication was "Death—a Necessary Concern for Nursing" [1968].)

My views were heightened by my commitment, if not my passion for or inner calling to advance (1) the discipline of nursing as a distinct profession with a more meaningful philosophical foundation for its science, congruent with its mission of caring-healing and health; (2) nursing's ethical covenant with society to sustain human caring and preserve human dignity, even when threatened; and (3) nursing's role in helping to sustain human dignity, humanity, and wholeness in the midst of threats and crises of life and death. All of these activities, experiences, questions, and processes transcend illness, diagnosis, conditions, setting, and so on. They were and remain enduring and timeless, and they exist across time and space and across changes in systems, society, civilization, and science.

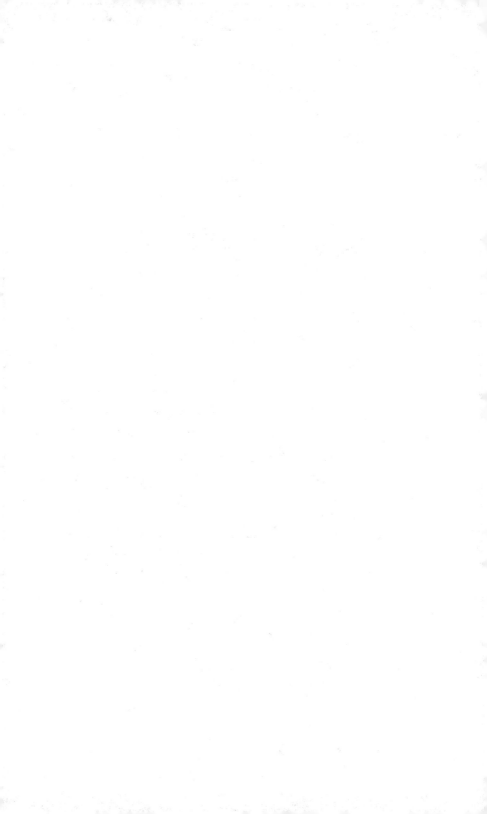

Appendix B

Overview of Jean Watson's Previous Caring Science Theory Books

My original (1979) work and the 2008 revision have expanded and evolved, generating a growing archive of publications, journals, other books, videos, and CDs, along with clinical-educational and administrative initiatives for transforming professional nursing. In explicating caring science as the foundation for nursing, we return to core values, core aspects of knowing beyond information, seeking perennial wisdom and truths that have been validated for centuries yet that somehow got lost during the rise of conventional Western culture and the dominant worldview of science and knowledge as objectivity, the be-all and end-all of life itself.

A series of my books on caring science and theory grounded in an expanded or basically timeless worldview followed; they have been translated into at least nine languages. My other major books based on theory–caring science that followed the original work include:

- *Nursing: Human Science and Human Care: A Theory of Nursing.* (1985). East Norwich, CT: Appleton-Century-Crofts. Reprinted/republished (1988). New York: National League for

Nursing. Reprinted/republished (1999). Sudbury, MA: Jones and Bartlett.

- *Postmodern Nursing and Beyond.* (1999). Edinburgh, Scotland: Churchill-Livingstone. Reprinted/republished New York: Elsevier.
- *Assessing and Measuring Caring in Nursing and Health Science.* (2002). New York: Springer (AJN Book of the Year award).
- *Caring Science as Sacred Science.* (2005). Philadelphia: F. A. Davis (AJN Book of the Year award).
- *Caring Science: Mindful Practice* (with K. Sitzman). (2012). New York: Springer.
- *Global Caring Literacy* (with S. Lee and P. Palmieri). (2017). New York: Springer.

Other caring-based books I coedited or coauthored are extensions of these works but are not discussed here (see, for example, Bevis and Watson [1989]; Watson and Ray, eds. [1998]; Chinn and Watson [1994]. Also see my website for complete citations of books and publications: www.watsoncaringscience.org.

Nursing: The Philosophy and Science of Caring (1979) provided the original core and structure for the Theory of Human Caring: Ten Carative Factors. At that time, these factors were identified as the essential aspects of caring in nursing, without which nurses may not have been practicing professional nursing but instead been functioning as technicians or skilled workers within the dominant framework of medical techno-cure science. This work has stood on its own as a timeless classic of sorts. It was not revised until 2008. The work has been kept alive through these two editions.

The present edition is an expanded and updated supplement of the original text, with completely new sections replacing previous sections while other sections that remain relevant have been included with minor revisions. I have been advised to retain the original text in this revision so that essential historical parts of ideas remain alive for future generations. Such continuity allows others to experience and study the historical evolution of ideas, theories, and the advancement of the discipline.

To provide the context for this evolution, I present a brief overview of the focus and content of the other books that continue to serve as background for my evolving work, all of which emerged from the original 1979 text.

For example, my second book, *Nursing: Human Science and Human Care: A Theory of Nursing*, expands on the philosophical, transpersonal aspects of a caring moment as the core framework. This focus places the theoretical ideas more explicitly within a broader context of ethics, art, and metaphysics as phenomena within which nursing dwells but which it often does not name, articulate, or act upon.

As has been pointed out in contemporary postmodern thinking, if a profession does not have its own language, it does not exist; thus it is important to name, claim, articulate, and act upon the phenomena of nursing and caring if nursing is to fulfill its mandate and raison d'être for society. This second theory text seeks to make more explicit the reality that if nursing is to survive in this millennium, it has to sustain and make explicit its covenant with the public. This covenant includes taking mature, professional responsibility for giving voice to, standing up for, and acting on its knowledge, values, ethics, and skilled practices of caring, healing, and health.

What was/is prominent in the second theory book is the explicit acknowledgment of the spiritual dimensions of caring and healing. There is further development of concepts such as the transpersonal, the caring occasion, the caring moment, and the "art of transpersonal caring" (Watson 1985, 67). Further, in this work, as reflected in the title, distinctions are made with respect to the context of human science in which nursing resides; for example:

- A philosophy of human freedom, choice, responsibility
- A biology and psychology of holism
- An epistemology that allows not only for empirics but also for the advancement of aesthetics, ethical values, intuition, personal

knowing, and spiritual insights, along with a process of discovery, creative imagination, evolving forms of inquiry

- An ontology of time *and* space
- A context of inter-human events, processes, and relationships that connect/are one with the environment and the wider universe
- A scientific worldview that is open. (Watson 1985, 16)

Thus a human science and human caring orientation differs from conventional science and invites qualitatively different aspects to be honored as legitimate and necessary when working with human experiences and human caring-healing, health, and life phenomena.

In this work one finds the first mention of "caring occasion," "phenomenal field," "transpersonal," and the "art of transpersonal caring," inviting the full use of self within a "caring moment" (Watson 1985, 58–72). The caring occasion/caring moment becomes transpersonal when "two persons [nurse and other] together with their unique life histories and phenomenal field [of perception] become a focal point in space and time, from which the moment has a field of its own that is greater than the occasion itself. As such, the process can [and does] go beyond itself, yet [it can and does] arise from aspects of itself that become part of the life history of each person, as well as part of some larger, deeper, complex pattern of life" (Watson 1985, 59).

The caring moment can be an existential-spiritual turning point for the nurse in that it involves pausing, choosing to "see"; it is informed action guided by an intentionality and a consciousness of how to *be* in the moment—fully present, open to the other person, open to compassion and connection, beyond the ego-control focus that is so common. In a caring moment, the nurse grasps the gestalt of the presenting moment and is able to "read" the field, beyond the outer appearance of the patient and the patient's behavior. The moment is "transpersonal" when the nurse is able to see and connect with the spirit of others, open to expanding possibilities of what can

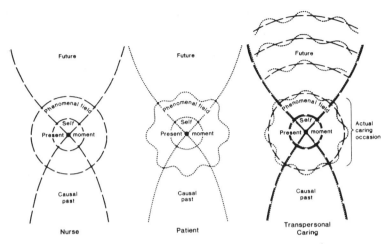

Transpersonal caring moment dynamics of the Human Caring Process. Reprinted with permission from Watson (1985).

occur. The foundation for this perspective is the wisdom in knowing and understanding that "we learn from one another how to be more human by identifying ourselves with others and finding their dilemmas in ourselves. What we all learn from it is self-knowledge. The self we learn about or discover is every self: it is universal. We learn to recognize ourselves in others" (Watson 1985, 59).

This human-to-human connection expands our compassion and caring and keeps alive our common humanity. This entire process deepens and sustains our shared humanity and helps avoid reducing another human being to the moral status of object (Watson 1985, 60).

This second book concludes with a sample of human science methodology as a form of caring inquiry. Transcendental phenomenology is discussed as one example of a human science–caring science experience of loss and grief experienced and researched among an aboriginal tribe in Western Australia. Poetry and artistic metaphoric expressions emerge within the "outback" research experience, using this extended methodology. Such an approach was consistent with the findings and experiences in this unique setting in that this methodology allowed for a "poetic" effect in articulating experiences as felt and lived, transcending their facts and pure descriptions (descriptive phenomenology).

Thus, the transcendent views were consistent with transpersonal dimensions and provided space for paradox, ambiguity, sensuous resonance, and creative expressions, going beyond the surface phenomenology (Watson 1985, 90–91). For example: "In other words, how could cold, unfeeling, totally detached dogmatic words and tone possibly teach the truth or deep meaning of a human phenomenon associated with human caring, transpersonal caring, and grief, and convey experiences of great sorrow, great beauty, passion, and joy. We cannot convey the need for compassion, complexity, or for cultivating feeling and sensibility in words that are bereft of warmth, kindness, and good feeling" (Watson 1985, 91). The result is poetizing; "it cannot be other than poetic" (Heidegger, quoted in Watson 1985, 98).

Indeed, during this era of evolving beyond conventional thinking, I served as dean of nursing at the University of Colorado (CU) in what is now the College of Nursing. I commissioned a prize-winning poet from CU's Boulder campus, Marilyn Krysl, to be in residence with us to "see" our clinical-medical world through her poetic eyes. I wanted her to help us go beyond the medicalized/clinicalized view of our humanity, whether faculty, student, patient, family, or administrator, and reconnect with the poetic beauty, yet poverty, of our humanity. Her publication *The Midwife and Other Poems on Caring* (1989) continues to be used by me and others around the world to awaken us to the wonders of our lifework and life world that are right under our noses but that we fail to see because of the medical lens we have accepted as the norm, especially in academic medical centers.

By inviting other ways of knowing and seeing, such as poetry and aesthetic methodology, caring science welcomes art, drama, theater, poetry, and all aesthetic creativity. This openness to celebrate, explore, and capture the depth and vicissitudes of our humanity is precisely what the world needs, what nursing and healthcare need, and what the soul of caring and healing needs, today more than ever.

An exemplar of methodology, such as transcendental phenome-nology, and having a poet in residence in an academic medical center, as far out as it may seem, allows for notions such as transcendence and going beyond the facts, so to speak; it invites a union of the humanities and art with science and spirituality, one of the perennial themes of my work. Finally, this history has helped me and contin-ues to help me build upon and further launch my ideas, expanding the foundation for a new/old worldview for the transformation of nursing and all of healthcare, of humanity-universe.

My third book, *Postmodern Nursing and Beyond* (1999), brought focus to the professional paradigm that is grounded in the ontology of relations and an ethical-ontological foundation before jumping to the epistemology of science and technology. The focus of this work was the need to clarify the ontological foundation of being-in-relation within a caring paradigm, the unity of mind-body-spirit/ field, going beyond the outdated separatist ontology of modern Era I medical-industrial thinking. In this book the spiritual and evolved energetic aspects of caring consciousness, intentionality, and human presence and the personal evolution of the practitioner became more developed. This evolution was placed within the emerging postmodern cosmology of healing, wholeness, and oneness that honors the unity of all.

This postmodern perspective attempts to project nursing and healthcare into the mid-twenty-first century, when there will be rad-ically different requirements for all health practitioners and entirely different roles and expectations between and among the public and healthcare systems (Watson 1999, xiii). Prominent in this text is an emphasis on the feminine yin energy needed for caring and healing, which nursing, other practitioners, and society alike are rediscov-ering because the dominant system is imbalanced with the arche-typal energy of yang, which is not the source of healing. Nursing serves as an archetype for healing and represents a metaphor for the deep yin healing energy that is emerging within an entirely dif-ferent paradigm. What is proposed is a fundamental ontological shift in consciousness, acknowledging a symbiotic relationship between humankind-technology-nature and the larger, expanding universe. This evolutionary turn evokes a return to the sacred core of humankind, inviting mystery and wonder back into our lives, work, and world. Such views reintroduce a sense of reverence for and openness to infinite possibilities. Emphasis is placed on the importance of ontological caring-healing practices, grounded in an expanded consciousness and intentionality that intersect with technological treatments of advanced medicine. In this work, Florence Nightingale's original blueprint for nursing is evident and embodies all the caring-healing nursing arts and rituals, rediscovered and honored for new reasons. Metaphors of *ontological archetype*, *ontological artist*, and *ontological architect* are used to capture the roles of and visions for nursing in this millennium/Era III medicine and nursing (Watson 1999, xiv–xv).

This book also introduces the notion of quantum caring, now further developed by collaboration with Tim Porter O'Grady and Kathy Malloch and their work in quantum leadership and global innovation at Arizona State University in Phoenix, leading to quantum caring leadership as a new turn that integrates the synthetic evolution of this work.

My theoretical book *Caring Science as Sacred Science* (2005) (which received an *American Journal of Nursing* Book of the Year award in 2006 in the category of research) expands further on the earlier works on caring. This work places Caring Science within an ethical-moral–philosophically evolved, scientific context, guided by the work of Emmanuel Levinas (1969, French) and Knud Logstrup (1997, Danish).

This book was both personal and theoretical, as it entered the holy and sacred personal life space of my own journey into suffering, loss, and deep mystical experiences. It provided me with the inner knowing; the deep, contemplative, introspective insight into and mystery of experiencing the non-physical, the cosmic field of love, beyond my ego self. During that journey, I actually became love. I was not in love, I was not loved; rather, I became a constellation of love, of universal energy dissolving into the infinite universal field. It is not something I or others can explain in conventional terms, but it is a knowing beyond knowing, a being beyond being, a oneness experience of the holy.

By using my own journey as an incentive, the caring science as sacred science work brought forth and uncovered another model of science that reintegrates metaphysics within the material physical domain and re-invites Ethics of Belonging (to the infinite field of Universal Cosmic Love) (Levinas 1969) as before and underneath *being by itself* alone—no longer separate from the broader universal field of infinity to which we all belong and to which we return from the earth plane.

Levinas's "Ethics of Face"—as in facing our own and others' humanity—is explored as a metaphor for how we deepen and sustain our humanity for survival of the human, in contrast to "totalizing" the human condition and cutting us off from the infinite source of life and the great cosmic field that unites us all. Logstrup's "ethical demand" brings forth the notion of "Ethics of Hand," in that he reminds us of the sovereign, unarticulated, often anonymous ethical demand that "we take care of the life which trust has placed in our hands" (Logstrup 1997, 18).

Caring Science as Sacred Science identifies these basic assumptions (Watson 2005, 56):

- The infinity of the human spirit and evolving universe
- The ancient and emerging cosmology of a unity consciousness of relatedness of all
- The ontological ethic of *belonging before our separate being* (Levinas 1969)
- The moral position of sustaining the infinity and mystery of the human condition and keeping alive the evolving human spirit across time, as in *facing and deepening our own and others' humanity* (Levinas 1969)

- The ethical demand that acknowledges that we hold another person's life in our hands; this sovereign expression of life is given to us before and beyond our control with expressions of trust, love, caring, honesty, forgiveness, gratitude, and so on; beyond ego fixations and obsessive feelings that are negative expressions of life (Logstrup 1997)
- The relationship among our consciousness, words, and thoughts and how they positively or negatively affect our energetic-transpersonal field of being, becoming, and belonging; thus, our consciousness affects our ability to connect, to "be in right relation" with source: the infinite universal cosmic field of LOVE.

In this evolved context of caring science, we can appreciate, honor, and face the reality that life is given to us as a gift; we are invited to sustain and deepen our own and others' humanity as our moral and ethical starting point for professional caring-healing. In Levinas's view, the "Ethic of Belonging" (to this universal field of Cosmic Love) becomes the first principle and starting point for any science, allowing ethics and metaphysics to be reunited with conventional science.

These views are not unlike Florence Nightingale's (1969) notion of natural healing processes, which draw upon spiritual dimensions that are the greatest source of healing. Indeed, it has been acknowledged in perennial philosophies and wisdom traditions across time, cultures, and a diversity of belief systems that the greatest source of healing is love. Thus, my book on sacred science brings a decidedly humble, holy, reverential dimension to the work of caring, making more explicit that we dwell in mystery and the infinity of Cosmic Love as the source and depth of all life.

As a Native American elder from the Ojibwe tribe instructed me, "We come from the spirit world and return to the spirit world/ source; when vulnerable, stressed, fearful, ill, and so forth, we all seek to return home, [to] that place that aligns us with our soul and our soul purpose." This is comparable to Nightingale's notion of putting the patient in the best condition for nature to heal, acknowledging that healing draws on nature and natural processes. In this framework it is acknowledged that we are working with the inner life forces, life energy, and the soul, if you will, of self and others and that we need to connect with the universal infinite field.

Appendix C

Charter of International Caritas Consortium (ICC)

As a result of recent national and international developments in the use of Caring Science Theory and Philosophy of Human Caring as a guide to transformative work in nursing scholarship, education, and practice, a gathering of invited professionals is emerging. These are committed professionals who are authentically being-doing and advancing the work in the world and who wish to convene to deepen the *Caritas Model*, share their activities, and learn from each other.

The group has named itself the International Caritas Consortium. Different institutions using this model host gatherings of these like-minded professionals upon invitation from me. All are from institutions in which the new caring-healing models are being implemented, along with selected others who are advancing Caring Science scholarship and practices. Anyone interested in participating can contact me at jean.watson@uchsc.edu. Additional information is on the Caritas Consortium website, www.caritasconsortium .org, and my website: www.uchsc.edu/nursing/caring.

INTERNATIONAL CARITAS CONSORTIUM (ICC) CHARTER

Purpose

The main purposes of this emerging International Caritas Consortium are:

1. To explore diverse ways to bring the caring theory to life in academic and clinical practice settings by supporting and learning from each other; and

2. To share knowledge and experiences so that we might help guide self and others in the journey to live the caring philosophy and theory in our personal/professional life.

The consortium gatherings will:

- Provide an intimate forum to renew, restore, and deepen each person's, and each system's, commitment and authentic practices of human caring in their personal/professional life and work;
- Learn from each other through shared work of original scholarship, diverse forms of caring inquiry, and model caring-healing practices;
- Mentor self and others in using the Theory of Human Caring to transform education and clinical practices;
- Develop and disseminate Caring Science models of clinical scholarship and professional excellence in the various settings in the world.

Membership

The participants of the Caritas Consortium are invited representatives of clinical and educational systems and/or selected individuals who are advancing the education, professional practice, and research of Caring Science/Human Caring Theory through their respective role and activities in the USA and various locations in the world.

Structure-Coordination: Core Caritas Coordinating Council (CCCC)

The Core Caritas Coordinating Council serves as a subgroup of the membership and functions as a coordinating and communicating body with the members. The core members will include:

- Dr. Jean Watson, founder of the original Theory of Human Caring, who serves as Chair/Honorary Chair;
- Selected representatives from original leadership member representatives from organizations/systems developing and advancing the model of caring theory and practices throughout their institution.

The council shall consist of six or fewer members, who will provide continuity and stability; coordinate the agendas; and provide leadership for emerging projects of the ICC.

Meetings

The ICC members and new invitees shall meet in the spring and fall of each year, per the sponsorship of member(s) who request to host the gathering. The host institution and its representatives shall serve as the primary organizing/agenda-setting body for the gathering in their institution, along with assistance from previous hosts, the Core Caritas Coordinating Council, and Dr. Watson.

Responsibilities/Activities for Gatherings

- Provide a safe forum to explore, create, renew self and system through reflective time-out.
- Share ideas, inspire each other, and learn together.
- Participate in use of Appreciative Inquiry whereby each member is facilitative of each other's work, each learning from others.
- Create opportunities for original scholarship and new models of caring-based clinical and educational practices.
- Generate and share multi-site projects in caring theory scholarship.

- Network for educational and professional models of advancing caring-healing practices and transformative models of nursing.
- Share unique experiences for authentic self-growth within the Caring Science context.
- Educate, implement, and disseminate exemplary experiences and findings to broader professional audiences through scholarly publications, research, and formal presentations.
- Envision new possibilities for transforming nursing and health care.

Appendix D

History of Hospital Sponsors—Sites of ICC

International Caritas Consortium History

23RD: OCTOBER 2017. Stanford Health Care (Palo Alto & San Mateo, CA)

22ND: OCTOBER 2016. Brigham & Women's Hospital (Boston, MA)

21ST: OCTOBER 2015. Gunderson Health System (Onalaska, WI)

20TH: OCTOBER 2014. St. John Hospital and Medical Center (MI)

19TH: OCTOBER 2013. Adventist Midwest Health (IL)

18TH: OCTOBER 2012. AtlantiCare Regional Medical Center (NJ)

17TH: APRIL 2012. WCSI, Boulder with participation with The Children's Hospital (CO)

16TH: MARCH 2012. First Global International Asian Pacific Caritas Consortium: Red Cross Hiroshima, College of Nursing, Hiroshima, Japan.

15TH: OCTOBER 2011. Michael E. DeBakey VA Medical Center (TX)

14TH: APRIL 2011. Winter Haven Hospital (FL)

13TH: OCTOBER 2010. Chesapeake Regional Medical Center (VA)

12TH: APRIL 2010. Kaiser Permanente, Antioch Medical Center (CA)

11TH: OCTOBER 2009. Wyoming Medical Center (WY)

10TH: APRIL 2009. Bon Secours, St. Francis Hospital (SC)

9TH: OCTOBER 2008. Jacksonville Baptist Medical Center (FL)

8TH: APRIL 2008. Scottsdale Healthcare (AZ)

7TH: OCTOBER 2007. Bon Secours, St. Mary's Hospital (VA)

6TH: MAY 2007. Scripps Memorial Hospital (CA)

5TH: OCTOBER 2006. Central Baptist Hospital (KY)

4TH: APRIL 2006. Inova Health System (VA)

3RD: OCTOBER 2005. Resurrection Medical Center (IL)

2ND: APRIL 2005. Baptist Health Miami (FL)

1ST: OCTOBER 2004. University of Colorado Health Sciences Center & The Children's Hospital (CO)

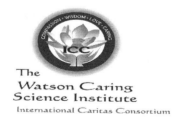

The
Watson Caring
Science Institute
International Caritas Consortium

Appendix E

Watson Caring Science Institute

About WCSI

The Watson Caring Science Institute (WCSI) is an international non-profit organization created to advance the philosophies, theories and practices of Human Caring, originated by Jean Watson, Distinguished Professor Emerita and Dean Emerita of University of Colorado Denver, College of Nursing, where she held the Endowed Chair in Caring Science at the University of Colorado Denver and Health Sciences Center. The Theory and Science of Human Caring seeks to restore the profound nature of caring-healing and bring the ethic and ethos of Love back into healthcare. Through an extended network of professional, clinical, and academic colleagues, the Institute will translate the model of Caring-Healing/Caritas into more systematic programs and services which can continue to transform healthcare, one nurse/one practitioner/one educator/one system at a time.

WCSI is dedicated to help the current healthcare system retain its most precious resource—competent, caring professional nurses—

while preparing a new generation of health professionals in a broader model of Caring Science. WCSI will help to ensure caring and healing for the public, reduce nurse turnover, and decrease costs to the system.

The Watson Caring Science Institute builds upon the lifetime background and global academic and clinical experiences of Dr. Jean Watson and her work in the field of Caring-Healing philosophy, theories, and practices. Dr. Watson has more than 30 years experience, with travels throughout the world. Working with expertise from WCSI faculty and over 300 trained Caritas Coaches®, Watson and her colleagues work to develop and implement the science, theories, and philosophies of caring and healing used by nurses and academic and clinical institutions internationally.

Program Overview

Dr. Watson and WCSI faculty focus on deeply personal, heart-centered, theory-guided Caritas Practices to transformative Caring–Healing professional Human Care models and modalities, attending to an energetic system-wide healing environment as Caritas field.

Caring Science expands and deepens the conventional model of medical science, offering a unitary world view of connectedness of all—thus Caring Science programs draw upon shared human spirit for creative new solutions, allowing for expanded views of humanity, of healing, of health.

The ten Caritas Processes® of Watson's theory provides language of phenomenon of human caring, which contributes to healing, wholeness, and human evolution, making new connections between human-to-human caring-love-healing and even peace in our world.

Programs

Dr. Watson and WCSI faculty:

- offer expertise with unique packages for keynotes, speaking, consultations, and workshops from WCSI faculty;
- provide intensive training programs in CaritasHeart™ Theory and Professional Practices;
- sponsor Global Consortia;
- sponsor and coordinate Watson Caring Science Global Associates with diverse countries;
- offer selected clinical-educational curriculum and research studies to meet diverse individual and system learning needs.

Each July, Dr. Watson conducts intense seminars for Watson Caring Science Postdoctoral Scholars based upon Caring Science as Sacred Science and emancipatory forms of inquiry.

Every October and April, the Caritas Coach Education Program® (CCEP)—a unique, six-month program offered by the Watson Caring Science Institute—is led by Jan Anderson, EdD, RN, AHN-BC, CCEP Director, Caritas Coach®, and HeartMath® Coach.

Every October, WCSI, in partnership with national caring science clinical educational systems, coordinate the International Caritas Consortium (ICC). The ICC is sponsored by clinical-academic organizations in various locations throughout the USA, implementing Caring Science in their settings as exemplars of this transformative work. Other Caritas consortia are now offered regionally in different parts of the country and other parts of the world.

WCSI 2.0

WCSI 2.0 means we are upgrading our Institute by consciously focusing on four distinctive parts which make up the whole: Legacy, Praxis, Education, and Research.

Education: WSCI 2.0 continues its dedication to help the current healthcare system retain its most precious resource—competent, caring, professional nurses. Our ambition is to prepare a new generation of health professionals in a broader model of Caring

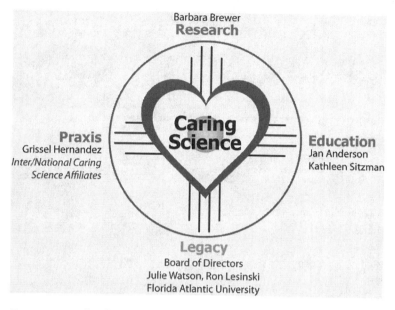

Barbara Brewer
Research

Praxis
Grissel Hernandez
*Inter/National Caring
Science Affiliates*

**Caring
Science**

Education
Jan Anderson
Kathleen Sitzman

Legacy
Board of Directors
Julie Watson, Ron Lesinski
Florida Atlantic University

Science. We do this by continuing to develop leaders through the unique 6- month Caritas Coach Education Programme (CCEP)™; the free, online Massive Open Online Course (MOOC), which combines the 10 Caritas Processes® with Mindful Practices of Thich Nhat Hanh (Vietnamese Buddhist Monk and Peace Activist). These are enhanced with online sessions with Dr. Watson. The MOOC course and WCSI education mission also extends to global caring science education for the public. Academic support is offered to colleges, university faculty, and students for caring science curriculum/pedagogies and authentic evaluation models. WCSI 2.0 overall educational aim is toward an evolving consciousness for moral community of caring/healing and health for all.

Praxis: Praxis, meaning informed moral practice. Our work is informed by the values, philosophy, theory, and ethic of human caring/healing. Praxis is distinguished from theory. WCSI 2.0 is dedicated to advancing professional theory-guided practice models of caring science. WCSI 2.0, with its international leaders, is dedicated to new clinical caring science praxis, criteria, and new standards to sustain human dignity, loving kindness, trusting relations, and a healing environment. The work is validated by new clinical Caritas outcomes. WCSI 2.0 National Caring Science Affiliates and partners are nationally recognized and designated as visionary exemplars of these futuristic transformative models of caring/healing healthcare for staff and patients/family/community.

Research: WCSI 2.0 recognizes that without research, nursing as a discipline is in danger of becoming obsolete and voiceless. We are on a mission to continue the research which captures and incorporates professional criteria of caring/healing (Caritas) with national outcomes, and new credentials are being developed based upon Caring Science/Heart Science (HeartMath.org), e.g., CaritasHealth™ programs. Research based upon caring science is leading to higher human caring/compassion standards for patient care and wider implications for our world and humanity. New ventures such as working in partnership with Press Ganey and gathering empirical data will support the theory and science of Human Caring, restoring the profound nature of caring-healing, and affirming the ethic and ethos of Love and Compassion back into healthcare.

Legacy: WCSI 2.0 is amalgamating the work of Dr. Jean Watson to sustain the robustness of the Institute and Caring Science for the future. Legacy work consists of creating a 'holding space' to gather, develop, and support the global community of Caring Science and foci in Caritas Praxis, Research, and Education strands in a coherent manner. This will enable Caring Science philosophy, values, theory, and practices to develop and grow, ensuring Watson Caring Science Institute will continue to carry out its original mission, programs, and purpose, now and into the future.

References

Abdellah, F. (1969). "The Nature of Nursing Science." *Nursing Research* 18 (5): 390–93.

Ackerknecht, E. H. (1968). *A Short History of Medicine.* New York: Ronald.

Aiken, L. H., H. K. Smith, and E. T. Lake. (1994). "Lower Mortality among a Set of Hospitals Known for Good Nursing Care." *Medical Care* 32: 771–87.

Alexander, E. (2012). *Proof of Heaven.* New York: Simon and Schuster.

American Nurses Association (ANA). (2015). *Nursing: Scope and Standards of Practice.* 3rd ed. Silver Spring, MD: ANA.

Aristotle. (2004). *The Nicomachean Ethics.* Trans. J.A.K. Thomson. London: Penguin.

Arman, M., A. Ranheim, K. Rydenlund, P. Rytterstrom, and A. Rehnsfeldt. (2015). "The Nordic Tradition of Caring Science: The Works of Three Theorists." *Nursing Science Quarterly* 28 (4): 288–96.

Arrien, A. (1993). *The Four Fold Way.* San Francisco: Harper.

Arrien, A. (2005). *The Second Half of Life.* Boulder: Sounds True.

Astin, J. (1991). *Remembrance.* CD. Santa Cruz, CA: Golden Dawn Productions.

Bache, C. (2001). *Transformative Learning.* Sausalito, CA: Noetic Sciences Institute.

Barks, C. (1997). *The Essential Rumi*. New York: Castle Books.

Barrett, E.A.M. (2002). "What Is Nursing Science?" *Nursing Science Quarterly* 15 (1): 51–60.

Barrett, E.A.M. (2017). "Again, What Is Nursing Science?" *Nursing Science Quarterly* 30 (2): 129–33.

Barrett, E.A.M., W. Cody, and J. Mitchell. (1997). "What Is Nursing Science? An International Dialogue." *Nursing Science Quarterly* 10 (1): 10–13.

Beardsley, E., and M. Beardsley. (1974). In *Metaphysics*, by Richard Taylor. 2nd ed. Englewood Cliffs, NJ: Prentice-Hall, ix.

Bell, J. S. (2016). *Twentieth Century Physics*. Oxford: Oxford University Press.

Benner, P. (1984). *From Novice to Expert: Excellence and Power in Clinical Nursing Practice*. Menlo Park, CA: Addison-Wesley.

Bent, K., J. Burke, A. Eckman, T. Hottmann, J. McCabe, and R. Williams. (2005). "Being and Creating Caring Change in a Healthcare System." *International Journal of Human Caring* 9 (3): 20–25.

Bernstein, R. J. (1983). *Beyond Objectivism and Relativism: Science, Hermeneutics, and Praxis*. Oxford: Basil Blackwell.

Berry, T. (1988). *The Dream of the Earth*. Sacramento: Sierra Club.

Bevis, E. O., and J. Watson. (1989). *Toward a Caring Curriculum*. New York: National League for Nursing.

Bigelow, C., ed. (2008). *The Pocket Ken Wilbur*. Boston: Shambhala.

Bjerg, S. (2002). "Jakob Knudsen: Totality through Life Experience." In R. Birkelund, ed., *Existence and Philosophy of Life*. Copenhagen: Gyldendal, 16–24.

Blegen, M. A., and T. A. Vaughn. (1998). "A Multisite Research of Nurse Staffing and Patient Occurrences." *Nursing Economics* 16 (4): 196–203.

Bohm, D. (1980). *Wholeness and the Implicate Order*. London: Routledge.

Bohm, D. (1989). *Quantum Theory*. Revised ed. New York: Dover.

Bohr, N. (1913). *On the Quantum Theory*. New York: Springer.

Bottorff, J. (1991). "Nursing: A Practical Science of Caring." *Advances in Nursing Science* 14 (1): 26–39.

Boyce, J. (2007). "Nurses Making Caring Work: A Closet Drama." PhD dissertation, Victoria University, Victoria, BC.

Boykin, A., and S. Schoenhofer. (2001). *Nursing as Caring: A Model for Transforming Practice*. New York: National League for Nursing.

Brewer, B., and J. Watson. (2015). "Evaluation of Authenticity of Human Caring in Professional Practices." *Journal of Nursing Administration* 45 (12): 1–6.

Broome, M. (2014). "Revisioning the Science of Nursing." *Nursing Outlook* 62: 159–61.

Buber, M. (1958). *I and Thou*. 2nd ed. New York: Scribner's.

Capra, F. (1975). *The Tao of Physics*. Boston: Shambhala.

Capra, F. (2013). *The Tao of Physics*. 5th ed. Boston: Shambhala.

Carr, W., and S. Kemmis. (1986). *Becoming Critical: Education, Knowledge, and Action Research*. London: Falmer.

Castaneda, C. (1998). *The Teachings of Don Juan*. New York: HarperPerennial.

Chinn, P. (2001). "Nursing and Ethics: The Maturing of a Discipline." *Advances in Nursing Science* 24 (2): v.

Chinn, P., and M. K. Kramer. (2008). *Integrated Theory and Knowledge Development in Nursing*. 7th ed. St. Louis, MO: Mosby.

Chinnery, A. (2001). "Asymmetry and the Pedagogical I-Thou." In S. Rice, ed., *Philosophy of Education Yearbook*. Urbana: University of Illinois Press, 189–91.

Chodron, P. (2005). *No Time to Lose*. Boston: Shambhala.

Conway, M. E. (1985). "Toward Greater Specificity in Defining Nursing's Metaparadigm." *Advances in Nursing Science* 7 (4): 73–81.

Cowling, W. R., III. (1994). "Unitary Knowing in Nursing Practice." *Nursing Science Quarterly* 6 (4): 201–7.

Cowling, W. R., III. (1999). "A Unitary-Transformative Nursing Science: Potentials for Transcending Dichotomies." *Nursing Science Quarterly* 12 (2): 132–37.

Cowling, W. R., III. (2000). "Healing as Appreciating Wholeness." *Advances in Nursing Science* 22 (3): 16–32.

Cowling, W. R., III, and E. Repede. (2010). "Unitary Appreciative Inquiry: Evolution and Refinement." *Advances in Nursing Science* 33: 64–77.

Cowling, W. R., III, M. Smith, and J. Watson. (2008). "The Power of Wholeness, Consciousness, and Caring: A Dialogue on Nursing Science, Art, and Healing." *Advances in Nursing Science* 31 (1): E41–E51.

Critchley, S., and R. Bernasconi. (2002). *The Cambridge Companion to Levinas*. Cambridge: Cambridge University Press.

Curtin, L. (2010). "Quantum Nursing." *American Nurse Today* 15 (9): 71–72.

Donaldson, S. K. (2002). "Nursing Science Defined in Less Than 10 Words." *Journal of Professional Nursing* 18 (2): 61, 112.

Donaldson, S. K., and D. M. Crowley. (1978). "The Disipline of Nursing." *Nursing Outlook* 26 (2): 113–20.

Dossey, B., and L. Keegan. (2008). *Holistic Nursing: A Handbook for Practice.* 6th ed. Sudbury, MA: Jones and Bartlett.

Dossey, B., and L. Keegan. (2014). *Holistic Nursing: A Handbook for Practice.* 5th ed. Sudbury, MA: Jones and Bartlett.

Dossey, B., and L. Keegan. (2015). *Holistic Nursing: A Handbook for Practice.* 7th ed. Boston: Jones and Bartlett.

Dossey, B., L. Keegan, and C. Guzzetta. (2000). *Holistic Nursing: A Handbook for Practice.* 3rd ed. Gaithersburg, MD: Aspen.

Dossey, B., L. Keegan, and C. Guzzetta. (2005). *Holistic Nursing: A Handbook for Practice.* 4th ed. Boston: Jones and Bartlett.

Dossey, L. (1991). *Meaning and Medicine.* New York: Bantam.

Dossey, L. (1993). *Healing Words, the Power of Prayer, and the Practice of Medicine.* San Francisco: Harper.

Dossey, L. (2004). *One Mind.* Carlsbad, CA: Hay House.

Duffy, J. (1992). "The Impact of Nurse Caring on Patient Outcomes." In D. Gaut, ed., *The Presence of Caring in Nursing.* New York: National League for Nursing, 395–405.

Duffy, J. (2002). "Caring Assessment Tools." In J. Watson, ed., *Instruments for Assessing and Measuring Caring in Nursing and Health Sciences.* New York: Springer, 131–48.

Duffy, J. (2003). "The Quality-Caring Model." *Advances in Nursing Science* 26 (1): 77–88.

Duffy, J., L. Hoskins, and R. F. Seifert. (2007). "Dimensions of Caring: Psychometric Properties of the Caring Assessment Tool." *Advances in Nursing Science* 39 (3): 1–12.

Dunlop, M. (1986). "Is a Science of Caring Possible?" *Journal of Advanced Nursing* 11: 661–70.

Dunphy, L. M., J. E. Winland-Brown, B. P. Porter, and D. Thomas. (2007). "Circle of Caring Model: A Transformative Model of Advanced Practice Nursing." In W. K. Cody, ed., *Philosophical and Theoretical Perspectives.* 2nd ed. Sudbury, MA: Jones and Bartlett, 285–94.

Emerson, R. W. (1982). *Ralph Waldo Emerson: Selected Essays.* New York: Penguin American Library.

Erikson, E. H. (1963). *Childhood and Society.* New York: Norton.

Erikson, K. (1999). *The Trojan Horse.* Vasa, Finland: Abo Akademi, Insitutionen for Vardvetenskap.

Erikson, K. (2002). "Caring Science in a New Key." *Nursing Science Quarterly* 15 (1): 61–65.

Fawcett, J. (1984). "The Metaparadigm of Nursing: Present Status and Future Refinements." *Image Journal of Nursing Scholarship* 16 (3): 84–89.

Fawcett, J. (2000). "The State of Nursing Science: Where Is the Nursing in the Science?" *Theoria: Journal of Nursing Theory* 9: 3–10.

Fawcett, J. (2002). "The Nurse Theorists: 21st-Century Updates—Jean Watson." *Nursing Science Quarterly* 15 (3): 214–19.

Foucault, M. (1972). *The Archaeology of Knowledge.* London: Tavistock.

Foucault, M. (1975). *The Birth of the Clinic: An Archaeology of Medical Perception.* Trans. A. M. Sheridan Smith. New York: Random/Vintage Books.

Foucault, M. (1977). *Power/Knowledge.* Edited by C. Gordon. New York: Pantheon.

Foucault, M. (1980). *Knowledge and Power.* New York: Pantheon.

Foucault, M. (1984). *The Foucault Reader.* Edited by P. Rabinow. New York: Pantheon.

Fox, M. (1985). *Illumination of Hildegard of Bingen.* Rochester, VT: Bear and Company.

Frampton, S., and P. Charmel, eds. (2009). *Putting Patients First: Best Practices in Patient-Centered Care.* 2nd ed. New York: Jossey-Bass.

Frankl, V. E. (1963). *Man's Search for Meaning.* New York: Washington Square Press.

Freire, P. (1996 [1972]). *Pedagogy of the Oppressed.* New York: Penguin.

Gadamer, H.-G. (1976). *Philsophical Hermeneutics.* Berkeley: University of California Press.

Gadamer, H.-G. (1977). *The Relevance of the Beautiful.* Edited by R. Bernasconi. Cambridge: Cambridge University Press.

Gadamer, H.-G. (1979). *Truth and Method.* London: Sheed and Ward.

Gore, A. (2006). *An Inconvenient Truth: The Planetary Emergency of Global Warming.* New York: Viking.

Gore, A. (2007). *An Inconvenient Truth: The Crisis of Global Warming.* New York: Viking.

Grace, P. J., D. G. Willis, C. Roy, and D. A. Jones. (2016). "Profession at the Crossroads: A Dialog Concerning the Preparation of Nursing Scholars and Leaders." *Nursing Outlook* 64: 61–70.

Greene, M. (1991). "Texts and Margins." *Harvard Educational Review* 61 (1): 25–39.

Hahn, Thich Nhat. (2003). *Creating True Peace.* New York: Free Press.

Halldorsdottir, S. (1991). "Five Basic Modes of Being with Another." In D. A.

Gaut and M. Leininger, eds., *Caring: The Compassionate Healer*. New York: National League for Nursing, 37–49.

Harman, W. W. (1990–91). "Reconciling Science and Metaphysics." *Noetic Science Review* 40: 5–10.

Harman, W. W. (1991). *A Re-examination of the Metaphysical Foundation of Modern Science*. Sausalito, CA: Institute of Noetic Sciences.

Harman, W. W. (1998). "What Are Noetic Sciences?" *Noetic Science Review* 47: 32–33.

Harvey, A. (2009). *The Hope: A Guide to Sacred Activism*. Melbourne, AR: Institute for Sacred Activism.

Hawkins, D. R. (2002). *Power vs. Force*. Carlsbad, CA: Hay House.

Heidegger, M. (1962). *Being and Time*. New York: Harper and Row.

Heidegger, M. (1971). "The Nature of Language." In M. Heidegger, ed., *On the Way to Language*. New York: Harper and Row, 14–20.

Heidegger, M. (1977). *Basic Writings: From Being and Time to the Task of Thinking*. New York: Harper and Row.

Heinlein, R. (1961). *Stranger in a Strange Land*. New York: Putnam.

Heisengber, W. (1930). *The Physical Principle of Quantum Theory*. New York: Dover.

Herbert, N. (1999 [1994]). In J. Watson, ed., *Postmodern Nursing and Beyond*. Edinburgh, UK: Churchill-Livingstone, 104.

Herman, K. (1993). "Reassessing Predictors of Therapist Competence." *Journal of Counseling Development* 72 (5): 29–32.

Hesse, H. (1951). *Siddhartha*. Trans. Hilda Rosner. New York: New Directions.

Hills, M., and J. Watson. (2011). *Creating a Caring Science Curriculum*. New York: Springer.

Hills, M., and J. Watson. (2012). *Creating a Caring Science Curriculum*. New York: Springer.

Holland, J. (2012). *Signals and Boundaries: The Building Blocks for Complex Adaptive Systems*. Boston: MIT Press.

Horvath, A. O., and B. D. Symonds. (1991). "Relation between Working Alliance and Outcome in Psychotherapy: A Meta-Analysis." *Journal of Counseling Psychology* 38 (2): 139–49.

Housden, R. (2005). *How Rembrandt Reveals Your Beautiful, Imperfect Self*. New York: Harmony Books.

Jarrin, O. (2006). "An Integral Philosophy and Definition of Nursing: Implications for a Unifying Theory of Nursing." Unpublished manuscript, July.

Jarrin, O. (2007). "An Integral Philosophy and Definition of Nursing." School of Nursing Scholarly Works 47. Accessed July 8, 2017. http://digitalcommons .uconn.edu/son_articles/47.

Joldersma, C. W. (2001). "Pedagogy of the Other: A Levinasian Approach to the Teacher-Student Relationship." In S. Rice, ed., *Philosophy of Education Yearbook*. Champaign: University of Illinois Press, 181–88.

Jonas, W. (2002). "Optimal Healing Relationships Research." Paper presented at the Samueli Institute Conference on Definitions and Standards in Healing Research. San Diego, CA, fall.

Kabat-Zinn, J., and M. Kabat-Zinn. (1997). *Everyday Blessings.* New York: Hyperion.

Kagan, Paula N., M. C. Smith, and P. L. Chinn. (2014). *Philosophies and Practices of Emancipatory Nursing: Social Justice as Praxis.* Oxford: Routledge.

Kagan, P. N., M. C. Smith, W. R. Cowling, and P. L. Chinn. (2009). "A Nursing Manifesto: An Emancipatory Call for Knowledge Development, Conscience, and Praxis." *Nursing Philosophy* 11: 67–84.

Kandinsky, W. (1977). *Concerning the Spiritual in Art.* New York: Dover.

Kaplan, S. H., S. Greenfield, and J. E. Ware. (1989). "Assessing the Effects of Physician-Patient Interactions on the Outcomes of Chronic Disease." *Medical Care* 27 (suppl. 3): S110–S127.

Kaptchuk, T. J., J. M. Kelley, L. A. Conboy, R. B. Davis, C. E. Kerr, E. E. Jacobson, I. Kirsch, R. N. Schyner, B. H. Nam, L. T. Nguyen, et al. (2008). "Components of Placebo Effect: Randomized Controlled Trials in Patients with Irritable Bowel Syndrome." *British Medical Journal* 3:336 (7651): 999–1003.

Kluckholn, C. M., H. A. Murray, and D. M. Schneider, eds. (1953). *Personality in Nature, Society, and Culture.* New York: Knopf.

Koerner, J. (2011). *Healing Presence: The Essence of Nursing.* New York: Springer.

Kornfield, J. (2002). *The Art of Forgiveness, Loving Kindness, and Peace.* New York: Bantam.

Kovner, C. T., and P. J. Gergen. (1998). "Nurse Staffing Levels and Adverse Events Following Surgery in US Hospitals." *Image: Journal of Nursing Scholarship* 30: 315–21.

Kreitzer, M. J. (2015). "Integrative Nursing: Application of Principles across Clinical Settings." Special issue on the Rambam-Mayo Collaboration, *Frontiers in Nursing* 6 (2). E0016.

Kreitzer, M. J., and M. Koithan, eds. (2014). *Integrative Nursing.* New York: Oxford University Press.

Krysl, M. (1989). *The Midwife and Other Poems on Caring.* New York: National League for Nursing.

Kuhn, T. (1970 [1962]). *The Structure of Scientific Revolutions.* 2nd ed. Chicago: University of Chicago Press.

Lafo, R. R., N. Capasso, and S. R. Roberts. (1994). "Introduction: Body and Soul: Contemporary Art and Healing." In R. R. Lafo, N. Capasso, and S. R. Roberts, eds., *Body and Soul: Contemporary Art and Healing.* Lincoln, NE: De Cordova Museum, 1–3.

Laing, R. D. (1965). *The Divided Self.* London: Pelican Book.

Laszlo, E. (1996). *The Whispering Pond: A Personal Guide to the Emerging Vision of Science.* Rockport, MA: Element Books.

Lather, P. (2007). *Getting Lost: Feminist Efforts toward a Double(d) Science.* New York: State University of New York Press.

Lather, P. (2010). *Engaging Science Policy: From the Side of the Messy.* New York: Peter Lang.

Lee, S., P. Palmieri, and J. Watson. (2016). *Global Caring Literacy.* New York: Springer.

Leininger, M. M. (1981). *Caring: An Essential Human Need.* Thorofare, NJ: Charles B. Slack.

Levin, D. (1983). "The Poetic Function in Phenomenological Discourse." In W. McBride and C. Schrag, eds., *Phenomenology in a Pluralistic Context.* Albany: State University of New York Press, 216–34.

Levinas, E. (1969). *Totality and Infinity.* Trans. A. Lingis. Pittsburgh: Duquesne University Press.

Linden, D. (1996). "Philosophical Exploration in Search of the Ontology of Authentic Presence." *Masters Abstracts International* 35 (1): 519.

Logstrup, K. (1997, Danish). *The Ethical Demand.* Minneapolis: Fortress.

Logstrup, K. (1997). *The Ethical Demand.* Notre Dame, IN: University of Notre Dame Press.

Luborsky, L., P. Crits-Cristophy, and A. T. McClellan. (1986). "Do Therapists Vary Much in Their Success? Findings from Four Outcome Studies." *American Journal of Orthopsychiatry* 56 (4): 501–12.

Macrae, J. A. (2001). *Nursing as a Spiritual Practice.* New York: Springer.

Malkin, J. (1992). *Hospital Interior Architecture: Creating Healing Environments for Special Patient Populations.* New York: Van Nostrand Reinhold.

Malloch, K., and T. Porter-O'Grady. (2010). *The Quantum Leader: Applications for the New World of Work.* Boston: Jones and Bartlett.

Martin, D. J., J. P. Garske, and K. M. Davis. (2000). "Relation of the Therapeutic Alliance with Outcome and Other Variables: A Meta-Analytic Review." *Journal of Consulting Clinical Psychology* 68 (3): 438–50.

Martinsen, K. (2006). *Care and Vulnerability*. Oslo, Norway: Akribe.

Marx Engels, K. (1976). *The German Ideology*. Moscow: Progress.

Maslow, A. H. (1968). *Toward a Psychology of Being*. Princeton, NJ: Van Nostrand.

McKivergin, D., and J. Daubernmire. (1994). "The Essence of Therapeutic Presence." *Journal of Holistic Nursing* 12 (1): 65–81.

McTaggert. L. (2002). *The Field: The Quest for the Secret Force of the Universe*. New York: HarperCollins.

Melange. (2009). "Quotations from Thomas Berry." *Melange* (blog). Accessed June 19, 2009. https://isiria.wordpress.com/2009/06/19/quotations-from -thomas-berry/.

Mitchell, S. (1994). *A Book of Psalms*. New York: HarperPerennial.

Moss, R. (1995). *The Second Miracle: Intimacy, Spirituality, and Consciousness*. Berkeley, CA: Celestial Arts.

Muff, J. (1988). "Of Images and Ideals: A Look at Socialization and Sexism in Nursing." In A. H. Jones, ed., *Images of Nursing: Perspectives from History, Art, and Literature*. Philadelphia: University of Pennsylvania Press, 197–224.

Munhall, P. (1993). "Unknowing: Toward Another Pattern of Knowing in Nursing." *Nursing Outlook* 4 (3): 125–28.

Myss, C. (1996). *Anatomy of the Spirit: The Seven Stages of Power and Healing*. New York: Harmony Books.

Nelson, J., and M. A. Hozak. (n.d.). "Relationship between HCAHPS Scores (Patient Experience) and Watson's Theory of Caring." Accessed January 15, 2017. http://www.nursinglibrary.org/vhl/bitstream/10755/621154/1/HC AHPSstudyposterv2April252016.pdf.

Newman, M. A. (1994). *Health as Expanding Consciousness*. Philadelphia: F. A. Davis.

Newman, M. A. (1997). "Experiencing the Whole." *Advances in Nursing Science* 20 (1): 34–39.

Newman, M. A. (2002). "The Pattern That Connects." *Advances in Nursing Science* 24 (3): 1–7.

Newman, M. A. (2003). "A World of No Boundaries." *Advances in Nursing Science* 26 (4): 240–45.

Newman, M. A., A. M. Sime, and S. A. Corcoran-Perry. (1991). "The Focus of the Discipline of Nursing." *Advances in Nursing Science* 14 (1): 1–6.

Newman, M. A., M. C. Smith, M. A. Dexheimer-Pharris, and D. Jones. (2008). "The Discipline of Nursing Revisited." *Advances in Nursing Science* 31 (1): E16–E27.

Newman, M. A., M. C. Smith, M. D. Pharris, and D. Jones. (2008). "The Focus of the Discipline Revisited." *Advances in Nursing Science* 31 (1): E16–E27.

Nightingale, F. (1969). Notes on Nursing: What It Is and What It Is Not. New York: Dover.

Okri, B. (1997). *A Way of Being Free.* London: Phoenix.

Okri, B. (2014). *The Age of Magic.* London: Head of Zeus.

Orlinsky, D. E., and K.I.L. Howard. (1985). "Therapy Process and Outcome." In S. Garfield and A. Bergin, eds., *Handbook of Psychotherapy and Behavior Change.* New York: John Wiley and Sons, 307–90.

Palmer, P. (1987). "Community, Conflict, and Ways of Knowing." *Magazine of Higher Learning* 19: 20–25.

Palmer, P. (2004). *The Violence of Our Knowledge: Toward a Spirituality of Higher Education.* 21st Century Learning Initiative. Kalamazoo, MI: Fetzer Institute.

Parse, R. R. (1998). *Human Becoming School of Thought.* Thousand Oaks, CA: Sage.

Parse, R. R. (2015). "Nursing Science or Is It the Science of Nursing?" *Nursing Science Quarterly* 28 (2): 101–2.

Parse, R. R. (2016). "Where Have All the Nursing Theories Gone?" *Nursing Science Quarterly* 29 (2): 101–2.

Parse, R. R., E. Barrett, M. Bourgeois, V. Dee, E. Egan, C. Germain, et al. (2000). "Nursing Theory–Guided Practice: A Definition." *Nursing Science Quarterly* 13 (2): 177.

Perkins, J. (2017). "Watson's Ten Caritas Processes Revisited through the Lens of Unitary Caring Science: Assessing the Sacred within Self." Unpublished manuscript.

Persky, G., J. Nelson, J. Watson, and K. Bent. (2008). "Creating a Profile of a Nurse Effective in Caring." *Nursing Administration Quarterly* 32 (1): 15–20.

Pesut, D. (2005). International Sigma Theta Tau President's Address. Indianapolis, IN, Sigma Theta Tau International.

Phillips, J. (2017). "New Rogerian Theoretical Thinking about Unitary Science." *Nursing Science Quarterly* 30 (3): 223–26.

Planck, M. (2016). *The Principle of Quantum Theory—From Planck's Quanta to Higgs-Bosom.* New York: Springer.

Plath, S. (1962). "Tulips." In *Ariel*, by Sylvia Plath. New York: Harper and Row, 160.

Popper, K. R. (1965 [1962]). *Conjectures and Refutations: The Growth of Scientific Knowledge*. New York: HarperTorchbooks.

Porter-O'Grady, T. (2010). "Leadership for Innovation: From Knowledge Creation to Transforming Healthcare." In T. Porter-O'Grady and K. Malloch, eds., *Innovation Leadership: Creating the Landscape of Healthcare*. Sudbury, MA: Jones and Bartlett, 1–32.

Porter-O'Grady, T., and K. Malloch. (2010). *Innovation Leadership: Creating the Landscape of Healthcare*. Sudbury, MA: Jones and Bartlett.

Porter-O'Grady, T., and K. Malloch. (2016). *The Leadership of Nursing Practice: Changing the Landscape of Health Care*. Cambridge, MA: Jones and Bartlett Learning.

Porter-O'Grady, T., and K. Malloch. (2017). *Quantum Leadership*. Philadelphia: Jones and Bartlett.

Quinn, J. F. (1989). "On Healing, Wholeness, and the Haelan Effect." *Nursing and Health Care* 10 (10): 553–56.

Quinn, J. F. (1992). "Holding Sacred Space: The Nurse as Healing Environment." *Holistic Nursing Practice* 6 (4): 26–35.

Quinn, J. F. (1997). "Healing: A Model for an Integrative Health Care System." *Advanced Practice Nursing Quarterly* 3 (1): 1–7.

Quinn, J. F. (2000). "Transpersonal Human Caring and Healing." In B. Dossey, ed., *Holistic Nursing: A Handbook for Practice*. 5th ed. Sudbury, MA: Jones and Bartlett, 91–100.

Quinn, J. F., M. Smith, C. Ritenbaugh, K. Swanson, and J. Watson. (2003). "Research Guidelines for Assessing the Impact of the Healing Relationship in Clinical Nursing." *Alternative Therapies in Health and Medicine* 9 (3) (suppl.): A65–A79.

Radin, D. (2015). "Meditation and the Non-Local Mind." *Explore: Journal of Science and Healing* 11 (2): 82–84.

Reason, P. (1988). *Human Inquiry in Action*. London: Sage.

Reason, P. (1993). "Reflections on Sacred Experience and Sacred Science." *Journal of Management Inquiry* 2 (3): 273–83.

Reed, P. G. (1997). "Nursing: The Ontology of the Discipline." *Nursing Science Quarterly* 10 (2): 76–79.

Reed, P. G., and N. B. Shearer. (2011). *Nursing Knowledge and Theory Innovation: Advancing the Science of Practice*. New York: Springer.

Reed, P. G., N. B. Shearer, and L. Nicholl. (2003). *Perspectives on Nursing Theory*. 4th ed. Philadelphia: Lippincott, Williams, and Wilkins.

Roach, M. S. (2002). *Caring, the Human Mode of Being: A Blueprint for the Health Professions*. 2nd ed. Ottawa: Catholic Health Association Press.

Rogers, M. E. (1970). *An Introduction to the Theoretical Basis of Nursing*. Philadelphia: Davis.

Rogers, M. E. (1988). "Nursing Science and Art: A Prospective." *Nursing Science Quarterly* 1 (3): 99–102.

Rogers, M. E. (1990). "Nursing: Science of Unitary, Irreducible Human Beings." In E.A.M. Barrett, ed., *Vision of Rogers' Science-Based Nursing*. New York: National League for Nursing, 5–11.

Rogers, M. E. (1992). "Nursing Science and the Space Age." *Nursing Science Quarterly* 6 (1): 27–33.

Rogers, M. E. (1994). "The Science of Unitary Human Beings: Current Perspectives." *Nursing Science Quarterly* 2 (1): 33–35.

Rolfe, G. (2011). "Practitioner-Centered Research: Nursing Praxis and the Science of the Unique." In P. G. Reed and N. B. Crawford Shearer, eds., *Nursing Knowledge and Theory Innovation: Advancing the Science of Practice*. New York: Springer, 59–74.

Rosenberg, S. (2006). "Utilizing the Language of Jean Watson's Caring Theory within a Computerized Clinical Documentation System." *CIN: Computers, Informatics, Nursing* 24 (1): 53–56.

Rotter, J. B. (1954). *Social Learning and Clinical Psychology*. Englewood Cliffs, NJ: Prentice-Hall.

Rumi, J. (2001a). *Hidden Music*. Trans. M. Mafi and A. Kolin. London: Thorsons/HarperCollins.

Rumi, J. (2001b). *The Glance: Rumi's Songs of Soul Meeting*. Trans. C. Barks. New York: Penguin Compass.

Ryan, L. (2005). "The Journey to Integrate Watson's Caring Theory with Clinical Practice." *International Journal of Human Caring* 9 (3): 26–30.

Samuels, M., and M. Land Rockwood. (2013). *Healing with the Arts*. Hillsboro, OR: Beyond Words.

Sarter, B. (1988). "Philosophical Sources of Nursing Theory." *Nursing Science Quarterly* 1 (2): 52–59.

Sartre, J. P. (1956). *Being and Nothingness*. New York: Philosophical Library.

Schlitz, M., E. Taylor, and N. Lewis. (1998). "Toward a *Noetic* Model of Medicine." *Noetic Science Review* 48: 45–52.

Schultz, W. C. (1967). *Joy: Expanding Human Awareness*. New York: Grove.

Senge, P., C. O. Scharmer, J. Jaworski, and B. S. Flowers. (2004). *Presence: An Exploration of Profound Change in People, Organizations, and Society*. New York: Doubleday, Random House.

Shambhala Training Glossary. (2011). Accessed January 18, 2017. http://www .glossary.shambhala.org.

Shattell, M. (2002). "Eventually It'll Be Over: The Dialectic between Confinement and Freedom in the Phenomenal World of the Hospitalized Patient." In S. Thomas and H. Pollio, eds., *Listening to Patients: A Phenomenological Approach to Nursing Research and Practice*. New York: Springer, 214–36.

Sheldrake, R. (1983). *A New Science of Life*. Los Angeles: Tarcher.

Sitzman, K., and J. Watson. (2012). *Caring Science: Mindful Practice*. New York: Springer.

Smith, M. C. (1992a). "Caring and the Science of Unitary Human Beings." *Advances in Nursing Science* 21 (4): 14–28.

Smith, M. C. (1992b). "Is All Knowledge Personal Knowing?" *Nursing Science Quarterly* 5 (1): 2–3.

Smith, M. C. (1994). "Arriving at a Philosophy of Nursing: Discovering? Constructing? Evolving?" In J. Kikuchi and H. Simmons, eds., *Developing a Philosophy of Nursing*. Thousand Oaks, CA: Sage, 43–60.

Smith, M. C. (1999). "Caring and the Science of Unitary Human Beings." *Advances in Nursing Science* 21 (4): 14–28.

Smith, M. C. (2010). "Nursing Theory and the Discipline of Nursing." In M. C. Smith and M. E. Parker, eds., *Nursing Theory and Nursing Practice*. 3rd ed. Philadelphia: F. A. Davis, 3–16.

Smith, M. C. (2013). "Caring and the Discipline of Nursing." In M. C. Smith, M. C. Turkel, and Z. R. Wolf, eds., *Caring in Nursing Classics: An Essential Resource*. New York: Springer, 1–8.

Smith, M. C. (2015a). "Marlaine Smith's Theory of Unitary Caring." In M. C. Smith and M. E. Parker, eds., *Nursing Theories and Nursing Practice*. 4th ed. Philadelphia: F. A. Davis, 509–19.

Smith, M. C. (2015b). "Nursing Theory and the Discipline of Nursing." In M. C. Smith and M. E. Parker, eds., *Nursing Theory and Nursing Practice*. 4th ed. Philadelphia: F. A. Davis, 1–18.

Smith, M. K. (2011 [1999]). "What Is Praxis?" *Encyclopaedia of Informal Education*. Accessed August 8, 2017. http://infed.org/mobi-what-is-praxis/.

Solomon, R. C., and K. M. Higgins. (1997). *A Passion for Wisdom: A Brief History of Philosophy.* Oxford: Oxford University Press.

St. Pierre, E. A. (2008). "Afterward: Decentering Voice in Qualitative Inquiry." In A. Jackson and L. Mazzei, eds., *Voices in Qualitative Inquiry.* London: Routledge, 221–36.

Stephenson, J., and T. Tripp-Reimer, eds. (1990). "Knowledge about Care and Caring." In *Proceedings of a Wingspread Conference,* February 1–3, 1989. Kansas City, MO: American Academy of Nursing.

Strupp, H. H., and S. W. Hadley. (1979). "Specific vs. Nonspecific Factors in Psychotherapy: A Controlled Study of Outcome." *Archives of General Psychiatry* 35 (10): 1125–36.

Swanson, K. (1999). "What Is Known about Caring in Nursing Research: A Literary Meta-Analysis." In A. S. Hinshar, S. Feetham, and J. Shaver, eds., *Handbook of Clinical Nursing Research.* Thousand Oaks, CA: Sage, 32–60.

Tarnas, Richard. (2006). *Cosmos and Psyche: Intimations of a New World View.* New York: Viking.

Teilhard de Chardin, P. (1955). *The Phenomenon of Man.* Toronto: R. P. Pryne.

Teilhard de Chardin, P. (1976). *The Phenomenon of Man.* New York: HarperPerennial.

Tolle, E. (1999). *The Power of Now.* Novato, CA: New World Library.

Tolle, E. (2003). *Stillness Speaks.* Novato, CA: New World Library.

Tolstoy, L. (1889a). *My Religion.* London: Walter Scott.

Tolstoy, L. (1889b [1968]). *The Wisdom of Tolstoy.* Trans. H. Smith. New York: Philosophical Library.

Tressolini, C. P., and Pew Fetzer Task Force. (1994). *Health Professionals Education and Relationship-Centered Care.* San Francisco: Pew Health Commission.

UNESCO. (2008). "Understandings of Literacy." *Education for All Global Monitoring Report.* Accessed January 30, 2016. www.Unesco.org.

van den Berg, J. H. (1966). *Psychology of the Sickbed.* Pittsburgh: Duquesne University Press.

Van Lommel, P. (2011). *Consciousness beyond Life.* New York: HarperCollins.

Vaughn, F. (1995). *Shadows of the Sacred: Seeing through Spiritual Illusions.* Wheaton, IL: Quest Books.

Walker, L. O., and K. C. Avant. (2005). *Strategies for Theory Construction in Nursing.* 4th ed. Englewood Cliffs, NJ: Pearson Education/Prentice-Hall.

Watson, J. (1968). "Death—a Necessary Concern for Nurses." In *Nursing Outlook*. New York: American Journal of Nursing Publication Co., 47–48.

Watson, J. (1979). *Nursing: The Philosophy and Science of Caring*. Boston: Little, Brown.

Watson, J. (1985). *Nursing Human Science and Human Care: A Theory of Nursing*. East Norwich, CT: Appleton-Century-Crofts.

Watson, J. (1996). "Watson's Theory of Trans-Personal Caring." In P. Hinton Walker and B. Neuman, eds., *Blueprint for Use of Nursing Models: Education, Research, Practice, and Administration*. New York: National League for Nursing Press, 141–84.

Watson, J. (1997). "The Theory of Human Caring: Retrospective and Prospective." *Nursing Science Quarterly* 10 (1): 49–52.

Watson, J. (1999). *Postmodern Nursing and Beyond*. Edinburgh, Scotland: Churchill-Livingstone; reprinted/republished New York: Elsevier.

Watson, J. (2001). "Post-Hospital Nursing: Shortages, Shifts, and Scripts." *Nursing Administration Quarterly* 25 (3): 77–82.

Watson, J. (2002a). *Assessing and Measuring Caring in Nursing and Health Science*. New York: Springer.

Watson, J. (2002b). "Intentionality and Caring-Healing Consciousness: A Practice of Transpersonal Nursing." *Journal of Holistic Nursing Practice* 16 (4): 12–19.

Watson, J. (2002c). "Love and Caring: Ethics of Face and Hand." *Nursing Administrative Quarterly* 27 (2): 197–202.

Watson, J. (2004a). "Caring Science." www.uchsc.edu/nursing/caring.

Watson, J. (2004b). "Commentary: Relational Core of Nursing Practice." *Journal of Advanced Nursing* 47 (3): 241–50.

Watson, J. (2005). *Caring Science as Sacred Science*. Philadelphia: F. A. Davis.

Watson, J. (2006). "Caring Theory as Ethical Guide to Administrative and Clinical Practices." *Nursing Administrative Quarterly* 30 (1): 48–55.

Watson, J. (2008a). "The International Caritas Consortium." www.caritasconsortium.org.

Watson, J. (2008b). *Nursing: The Philosophy and Science of Caring*. Boulder: University Press of Colorado.

Watson, J. (2008c). "The Watson Caring Science Institute." www.watsoncaringscience.org.

Watson, J. (2009). "Being Present: A Caring Moment." In S. Frampton and P. Charmel, eds., *Putting Patients First*. 2nd ed. New York: Jossey-Bass, 13–14.

Watson, J. (2012). *Human Caring Science.* Sudbury, MA: Jones and Bartlett.

Watson, J. (2014). "Social/Moral Justice from Caring Science Cosmology." In P. N. Kagan, M. C. Smith, and P. L. Chinn, eds., *Philosophies and Practices of Emancipatory Nursing: Social Justice as Praxis.* Oxford: Routledge, 64–70.

Watson, J. (2017). "Global Caritas Literacy." In S. Lee, P. Palmieri, and J. Watson, eds., *Global Caring Literacy.* New York: Springer, 3–11.

Watson, J. (In press). "Integrative Nursing—Unitary Healing Principles." In M. J. Kreitzer and J. Koithan, eds., *Integrative Nursing,* 2nd ed. New York: Oxford University Press.

Watson, J., and B. Brewer. (2015). "Caring Science Research, Criteria, Evidence, Measurement." *Journal of Nursing Administration* 45 (5): 235–36.

Watson, J., and R. Browning. (2012). "Caring Science Meets Heart Science: A Guide to Authentic Caring Practice." *American Nurse Today* 7 (8): 3. http://www.Americannursetoday.com/Popups/ArticlePrint. aspx?id=110508.

Watson, J., T. Porter-O'Grady, S. Horton-Deutsch, and K. Malloch. (2018 in press). "Quantum Caring Healthcare Leadership: Integrating Quantum Leadership with Caring Science." *Nursing Science Quarterly.*

Watson, J., and M. C. Smith. (2002). "Caring Science and the Science of Unitary Human Beings: A Transtheoretical Discourse for Nursing Knowledge Development." *Journal of Advanced Nursing* 37 (5): 452–61.

Watson, J., M. Smith, and R. Cowley. (2018 in press). "Unitary Caring Science: Disciplinary Evolution of Nursing." In W. Rosa, S. Horton-Deutsch, and J. Watson, eds., *Handbook for Caring Science.* New York: Springer.

Weber, R. (1986). *Dialogues with Scientists and Sages: The Search for Unity.* London: Routledge.

Werley, H. H., and N. M. Lang, eds. (1988). *Identification of the Nursing Minimum Data Set.* New York: Springer.

Whitehead, A. N. (1985). *Science and the Modern World.* Cambridge: Cambridge University Press.

Wilber, K. (1996). *A Brief History of Everything.* Boulder: Shambhala.

Wilber, K. (1998). *The Essential Ken Wilber.* Boston: Shambhala.

Wilber, K. (2000) *Sex, Ecology, Spirituality.* Boston: Shambhala.

Wilber, K. (2001a). *A Theory of Everything.* Boston: Shambhala.

Wilber, K. (2001b). http://wilber.shambhala.com/html/misc/haberman/.

Williamson, M. (2002). *Everyday Grace.* New York: Riverhead.

Woolf, V. (1938). *Three Guineas.* London: Hogarth.

Yalom, I. D. (1975). *Theory and Practice of Group Psychotherapy.* 2nd ed. New York: Basic Books.

Young, S. (2006). Accessed January 12, 2017. http://shinzen.org.

Zukav, G. (2013 [1979]). *The Dancing Wu Li Masters.* New York: HarperCollins.

Index

Page numbers in italic indicate illustrations.

Laing, R. D., 9, 109
Lane, Mary Rockwood, 107
language, to express Caritas Processes, 133–35
Lather, Patti, on wise knowing, 61–62, 63
learning, 55, 68, 140
Levinas, Emmanuel, 47, 45, 60, 101, 164, 165; on Ethic of Belonging, 13–14, 40–41, 142, 166
life-death circle, 146–47
light, and energy, 53
Linden, Danielle, 92
listening, 84; presence and, 93, 97
literacy, 43, 70; Caritas Presence, 98–99; Caritas-Veritas, 48, 49, 50, 55, 56, 66, 71, 72–75, 82–85; critical, 75–79; moral, 69, 87
Logstrup, Knud, 164, 165
love, 42, 116, 148; becoming, 164–65; and caring, 45–46; as Caritas value, 47–48, 49
loving-kindness, 136, 138
loving touch, 84

Malloch, Kathy, 164
Maori, 21
marches, public, 107
Massive Open Onlne Course (MOOC), Caritas Processes, 178
Maya calendar, 143–44
Mazer, Susan, 106, 112
medical praxis, 21
metal epoch, 143–44
meta-paradigm thinking, 32–33, 34
meta-philosophy, of Unitary Caring Science, 150–51
metaphysics, 5, 9, 11–12, 141, 143, 145; circle of life-death, 146–47; and science, 36, 61; spiritual in, 147–48; of unitary caring science, 148–49; Western, 149–50
Midwife and Other Poems on Caring, The (Krysl), 162
mind-body-spirit, unity of, 163
Mindful Practices of Thich Nhat Hanh, 178
minister (humanity), 135, 140
miracles, 55
moral actions, 73
moral foundation, 10, 49; of nursing practice, 21–22

morality, moral values, xix, 25, 50, 76, 87, 101; self and, 78–79
moral literacy, 69, 74–75
moral practice, 22
Munhall, Patricia, 62

National Caring Science Affiliates, 179
National Caring Science Systems, 119
National Institute of Nursing Research (NINR), 19
nature, as healing, 167
Newman, Margaret, 53, 114; "The Focus of the Discipline Revisited," 33; Theory of Expanding Consciousness, 35
New Story, 7–8, 18–19
New Zealand, Nursing Praxis, 21
Nightingale, Florence, 23, 100, 103, 112, 164; on healing, 114, 166–67
NINR. See National Institute of Nursing Research
nurses: as ontological archetype, 103–5
nursing, 8, 37, 46, 103; academic, 153–55; Caritas-Veritas Literacy in, 56, 82–85; as discipline, xvi, xviii, 64; disciplinary consciousness in, 31–32; integrative, 113–17; praxis, 21–22; theories of, 68–69; as unified whole, 33–34; Unitary Caring Science in, 64–66; wholeness, consciousness, and caring, 42–43
Nursing: Human Science and Human Care: A Theory of Nursing, concepts in, 159–63
Nursing: The Philosophy and Science of Caring (Watson), 158–59
"Nursing and Ethics: The Maturing of a Discipline" (Chinn), 37
Nursing Praxis (journal), 21
Nursing Professional Framework, 120
nursing science, 17–18; major paradigms in, 32–33
nursing skills, in Caritas-Veritas praxis, 85
nurture (relationship), 135, 139

O'Grady, Tim Porter, 164
Omega point, 47, 101, 149
oneness, xvi, 32, 36
oneness-wholeness, 67
online learning, 68
ontological caring literacy, 43

Theoria, 16–17
theory, 16–17; of nursing, 68–69; unifying, 37–41
Theory of Expanding Consciousness, 35
Theory of Human Becoming, 35
Theory of Transpersonal Caring, 50–54
Theory of Truth, 15; in Unitary Caring Science, 16–19
therapeutic presence, 91
therapeutic touch (TT), 84
Thich Nhat Hanh, 178
totalizing, of humanity, 101–2
touch, 84
transcendental phenomenology, 161–62
transpersonal, 50
transpersonal caring, 63, 91, 145–46, 149, 159; presence in, 93, 94–95; theory of, 50–54
Transpersonal Caring Consciousness, 53–54
transpersonal caring moments, 41–42, 44, 145–46, 160–61
Transpersonal Caring Science (TCS), 35, 38, 42, 79
transpersonal dimensions, 162
transpersonal self, 139
Transpersonal Theory of Human Caring (Transpersonal Caring Theory), xix–xx, 79
travel, and human connection, 144–45
treatment, 6
trust (transpersonal self), 6, 134, 139
truth, 10; theories of, 15–16. *See also* Veritas
truth-love, 6

Unitary Being, 16
Unitary Caring, 39–40; disciplinary matrix of, 64–65
Unitary Caring Science (UCS), xv–xvii, xviii, xix–xx, 6, 7, 8, 31, 39–40, 42, 73, 104, 138, 142; Caritas Literacy in, 83–85; and Ethic of Belonging, 60–66; and integrative nursing, 116–17; literacy in, 75–79; as meta-philosophy, 150–51; metaphysics and, 148–49; in nursing education, 65–69; and science, 87–88
unitary field, 142
Unitary Transformative, 31
Unitary Transformative (UT) paradigm, 33, 34, 42
unitary transformative paradigm, 6

unitary worldview, 143
unity, 60
unity of consciousness, 50, 61
Universal Cosmic Love, 14, 60, 142, 165, 166
universal humanity, 71
Universal Love, 41, 97, 101
universal unitary principles, 115
universe, sacred context, 11
University of Arizona, Integrative Fellowship Program, 113
University of Colorado, 106; academic nursing, 153–54; School/College of Nursing, 154–55, 162
University of Colorado Anschutz Medical Center, 154
University of Minnesota, Center for Spirituality and Healing, 113

values, 83, 111; of Caritas, 47–50, 54; Caritas-Veritas, 63–64; and Caritas-Veritas literacy, 78–79; moral-ethical, 25, 37; study of, 9–10
Veritas, 7, 45, 58, 63, 72, 73, 83; art in, 101, 111; moral foundation of, 10, 52; as praxis, 22–23
Veritas Aequitas, 10
veterans, soul care, 102
Virginia Commonwealth University Hospital (Richmond), 103–4; Watson Room, 122
virtue, 72

Watson Caring Science Institute (WCSI), 107, 119; programs, 176–79; purpose of, 175–76; Reflective Caritas Cards, 134
Watson Caring Science Postdoctoral Scholars, 177
Watson Rooms, 103–4, 122
Whitehead, Alfred North, 51, 143
wholeness, 42
whole person, dignity of, 21–22
Wilber, Ken, 62, 150
Winterhaven Hospital (Fla.), Caritas visualizing, 121
wise knowing, wisdom, xx, 61–62, 63
Women's March on Washington, 107

yin and yang, 104, 163

Zukav, Gary, 53